THROUGH
fire
& sea

⚓

ADVENTURES ON THE MERCY SHIP — A FAMILY'S
JOURNEY TO THE WORLD'S FORGOTTEN POOR

Marilyn Meyers

Through Fire & Sea: Adventures on the Mercy Ship

Copyright ©2007 Marilyn Meyers
Second Edition 2007
All rights reserved
Printed in Canada
International Standard Book Number: 978-1-897213-33-9

Published by:
BayRidge Books
Willard & Associates Consulting Group
1-1295 Wharf Street, Pickering, Ontario, L1W 1A2
Tel: (416) 573-3249   Fax (416) 226-4210
E-mail: info@bayridgebooks.com
www.bayridgebooks.com

Written by Marilyn Meyers
Cover Design by Salt Creative Goup Inc.
Printed at Essence Publishing, Belleville, Ontario

This book or parts thereof may not be reproduced in any form without prior written permission of the publishers.

Scripture references taken from THE MESSAGE Copyright ©1993, 1994, 1995, 1996, 2000, 2001, 2002. Used by permission of NavPress Publishing Group. • Scriptures marked NIV are from The Holy Bible, New International Version. Copyright © 1973, 1978, 1984 International Bible Society. Used by permission of Zondervan Publishing House. All rights reserved.

Library and Archives Canada Cataloguing in Publication

Meyers, Marilyn, 1957-
Through fire & sea : adventures on the Mercy Ship : a family's journey to the world's forgotten poor / Marilyn Meyers.

ISBN 978-1-897213-33-9

1. Meyers family. 2. Mercy Ships. 3. Charities, Medical. 4. Hospital ships.
2. 5. Christian biography--Canada. 6. Africa, West--Biography.

I. Title. II. Title: Through fire and sea.

HV687.M49 2007   362.1   C2007-903150-1

BayRidge
B O O K S

Dedicated to:

My husband Bruce
Prince and shipmate,
Who honours me with pure devotion.

My children Brandon, Chadwick and Jillian
Three valiant sailors,
Whose shining lives are emblazoned
on my heart for eternity.

My Heavenly Captain
Navigator and Refiner of my soul,
Who saturates the pages of my life with
extravagant love and mercy.

Acknowledgements

A group of generous Norwegians offered the couples of the *Anastasis* a retreat in the countryside. There in the rugged terrain and beauty of Norway, creativity that lay dormant awoke, along with the vague seed of this book.

A year later in the upper loft of a skylight restaurant in Scotland, Bruce and I celebrated an anniversary in yet another corner of the world. That day Bruce watered the seed with courage and belief, something I failed to muster within myself. The seed grew larger.

In the second year of our return from the Mercy Ship, I sat with my laptop overlooking the vestige of land which we now call home. The seed took root and finally broke through the surface of the soil as I began the story. The tiny exposed shoots battled against the elements of self-doubt.

Without the encouragement of audiences where I speak, friends and family prodding me along, the story would have remained unfinished on my laptop. A strong editorial team brought unique finishing touches and the tender shoots grew into a book.

Sincere thanks to my editorial team for their hard work and unique perspectives:

- To Beth Wilton, whose friendship and life dedicated to the poor of Winnipeg's north end never ceases to inspire and challenge me, for her insightful thoughts, sound wisdom and questions on technical ship terms.

- To Steve Crewson, our former youth pastor, for his male perspective, his gentle honesty, theological expertise and persistence in editing through busy, hard times.
- To Lorraine McDonald, my boss and fellow crewmember, for her professional editing of grammar and sentence structure, checking for accuracy, but most of all for nudging me when I'd stopped nurturing the growth of the book.
- To Bruce Meyers, my teacher husband, for his macro and micro-editing, encouragement and patience. His strong belief in me took me over the abyss of self-doubt and fear to the completion of this project.

Finally, I wish to acknowledge Mrs. Haufschild, my grade five teacher, who believed I would grow up to be a writer. Her words impacted me in grade school like none other. I grew up, and I do love to write!

Special thanks to my children for living the story and most of all to my Heavenly Father, the writer and editor of my soul.

contents

PART ONE - Through the Fire

Chapter 1	Sunken Hopes	4
Chapter 2	Dream Sparks	9
Chapter 3	Tests in the Wilderness	20
Chapter 4	Soul Thirst	27
Chapter 5	Silence in the Crib	37
Chapter 6	Bread of Adversity	41
Chapter 7	Beauty from Ashes	47
Chapter 8	Currier & Ives	57
Chapter 9	Embers of a Dream	64
Chapter 10	Smoky Kiln	71
Chapter 11	Death at the Crossroads	79
Chapter 12	Triumph in Trinidad	85
Chapter 13	Call Aboard	95

PART TWO - Through the Sea

Chapter 14	Painted Porthole	106
Chapter 15	Forth to the Sea	115
Chapter 16	Fires, Riots and Pirates	123
Chapter 17	Steel Scars	129
Chapter 18	Floating Village	135
Chapter 19	The Homecoming	143
Chapter 20	Weeping with the Wounded	153
Chapter 21	Hope and Healing	161
Chapter 22	Clay Vessels of Mercy	167
Chapter 23	Cabin to Compound	175
Chapter 24	Humbled by the Poor	187
Chapter 25	Honoured by the Rich	193
Chapter 26	School of Mercy	203
Chapter 27	Mercy Hands	213
Chapter 28	Mercy for Missionaries	219
Chapter 29	Remember the Poor	225
Chapter 30	Reflections in the Sea	235

THROUGH fire & sea

⚓

ADVENTURES ON THE MERCY SHIP — A FAMILY'S
JOURNEY TO THE WORLD'S FORGOTTEN POOR

Marilyn Meyers

*Water and fire succeed
The town, the pasture and the weed.
Water and fire deride
The sacrifice that we denied.
Water and fire shall rot
The marred foundations we forgot,
Of sanctuary and choir.
This is the death of water and fire.*

T. S. Eliot – Little Gidding

PART ONE
Through the fire

When you walk through the fire, you will not be burned; the flames will not set you ablaze.

Isaiah 43:2

1
Sunken Hopes

> *Hope deferred makes the heart sick,*
> *but a longing fulfilled is a tree of life.*
> Proverbs 13:12

Briefly I left my husband's bedside to answer the knock at the door. "It's the doctor's office on the phone for you," she whispered in a low voice. I quickened my pace to the small phone booth down the hall.

"Your husband's results are positive for Hepatitis C," stated the nurse flatly. Stunned, I stood silent for several long seconds. My thoughts raced searching for a reasonable path to understanding.

"What does that mean?" I stammered. "Does he have the disease?" The words stumbled out making me feel rather foolish. She repeated her original statement adding that I would need to get further information from the doctor. It still made no sense.

Dazed, I returned to the chair beside Bruce's bed. His face seemed even paler than before I had left. My thoughts immediately turned to the children and how I would break this news about their father's illness. That could wait, I decided as I rounded them

Chapter One

up to set out for the dining hall across the lush, tree-covered grounds of East Texas.

Hours later the doctor's news began to sink into my tattered spirit. We were finally living at the edge of our dream—a dream that spanned 12 years of preparation. Now at age 38, my healthy, vibrant husband was stricken with a mysterious, incurable, lifelong disease. And we were over a thousand miles from home.

When I first broke the doctor's news of Hepatitis C to Bruce, he was too sick to care or understand. I felt anxious and confused as I attempted to come to grips with the news alone. The companionship of my classmates in the Crossroads Discipleship Training School brought me a measure of comfort and assurance. All of us had sacrificed much to be there, preparing for a life in missions. Some rallied around me while others warmly visited Bruce's bedside. One friend began to research the disease from the Internet which in 1997 had become a new, resourceful tool. Together we huddled curiously around the blue glowing light of Chris's laptop in the family lounge.

We discovered that Hepatitis C is a virus that infects the liver. Inflammation or swelling of the liver can lead to cirrhosis, the leading cause of liver disease. Symptoms could include nausea, vomiting, joint and muscle aches, abdominal pain and weight loss. Bruce seemed to exhibit everything and more! I dared not speculate what all this news meant for our future. Bruce and I had finally reached an exciting crossroads in our lives. Surely nothing would stand in our way now!

The violent retching continued for several days. Between classes, I ran to our dorm room to check on him. I redampened the terry cloth and laid it lovingly on his blazing forehead. He moaned softly with no consciousness of my presence.

I knew he should probably be in a hospital bed tended to by doctors and nurses, but we were Canadians temporarily living in Texas and had no health plan in the USA. In our somewhat hasty departure we'd been unable to obtain insurance. When we'd inquired about coverage, openly explaining our plans to government officials, our Ontario Health Insurance Plan had been cut off immediately after our departure. Although medical costs in the US could wipe out people's life savings, of which we had little, we had chosen to leave anyway. What could possibly happen? We had assured ourselves that our health was in God's hands and then stepped out in faith. Now the finger of accusation for our foolishness seemed to point in our faces.

I felt at a loss to assess the situation properly. How much longer could I wait this out? Surely he will recover soon. Suddenly Bruce roused, gasping and moaning. Reaching for the bucket, he dry-heaved hideously. His pale face looked gaunt and haggard, his huge eyes bleary and distant. Laying his head slowly back on the pillow, he quieted down once again. My fears heightened and I wept softly for the suffering of the man I had loved deeply for 12 married years.

Far from home and alone at the helm of our family, the burden felt heavy and unbearable. Our three children seemed oblivious to the severity of it all. Happily, they engaged in play with other children on the Mercy Ships International training base. They knew their dad had become quite ill since he returned from his emergency knee operation in Ontario. Thrilled to have him back, it mattered little what state he came in. They simply prayed, left the matter to God and returned to play with their new, exciting friends.

Nursing a sick husband became my first overriding concern.

Chapter One

I grew more overwhelmed, stretched in my roles of nurse, mother and student. Part of that time also included work duties. Assigned hospitality duty for the weekly visiting speakers, I laundered their clothes and cleaned their room in the Anchorage Hotel on the base. Between speakers' visits, the spacious room was left clean and empty.

One day, pouring out my fears to God in that empty room, I slumped to my knees beside the king-sized bed. I had been learning about the power of intercessory prayer in our lectures. On Bruce's behalf I prayed fervently, earnestly for God to heal him; losing all sense of time, the minutes or hours slipped by. Eventually the need for prayer ceased and I felt light and hopeful. I rose and ran out of the ranch-style hotel. Stopping for no one, I headed across the sprawling base to our dorm room. Breathlessly I opened the door. As I'd hoped, Bruce sat peacefully alert on the edge of the bed. He focused and smiled at me. "Hi dear," he said sweetly.

"Hi lover," I responded with great relief in my voice. "You look so much better!"

"Lynn brought me some Gatorade and I feel a lot better," he offered weakly. A concerned classmate had suspected dehydration. Like a wilted flower, it had watered and revived him. Finally, the breakthrough I had prayed for. Hopefully, the road to recovery and missions lay ahead.

Days later, weak but walking, Bruce and I made the trip to the doctor in Tyler, Texas. Unaware of the full ramifications, our new US doctor broke the news matter-of-factly, "It's too dangerous for you to leave the country."

Because of his acute Hepatitis C, our mission trip to Trinidad was out of the question. Without this assignment to a developing country, we could not complete our training requirements for service with Mercy Ships. Without complete training, we could not fulfill the dream of sailing to the poor on the *Anastasis*.

We were so close. Surely we would not have to suffer and endure this colossal disappointment in our lives, not after all we'd been through already! The crushing thought of returning home to Ontario empty-handed after giving up everything was a grief far beyond my strength to bear. I refused the cruel thought.

Later, the magnitude of it all struck me. We had nothing to turn back to at home, nothing to go forward to in a mission career and in bed lay a husband with an incurable disease. How dreadfully ironic that we aspired to join a mission organization offering hope and healing to the poor and now we ourselves were deeply, desperately in need of both!

Deep wrenching sobs—the kind that leaves one exhausted for hours—overtook me in the darkness of the family dorm. Our dream of sailing to the poor sank that night.

But like Mercy Ships, this also is a story of hope and healing.

2
Dream Sparks

> *There is surely a future hope for you,*
> *and your hope will not be cut off.*
> *Proverbs 23:18*

Friends teased me about the color of my bright, spring green Ford Mustang. But in 1983 it had become my greatest asset and the odd colour had grown on me. With the trunk jammed full, and the back seat filled with my few earthly belongings, I drove out of Winnipeg for the last time. The city skyscrapers spiking up from the flat prairie earth slowly faded away as I glanced in my rear-view mirror. I knew assuredly that deep sadness and longing would follow. But for now I would look forward and enjoy the long trip ahead.

Before crossing the Ontario border, I checked on the forest of green house plants in the front seat beside me. I had lovingly nurtured each plant for four years and couldn't bear to leave them behind. I wondered if they would even survive the fierce, deep winter chill of my trek through Northern Ontario. Turning up the heater full blast, it barely restrained the -27 Celsius temperature from frosting up the windshield. Onward I journeyed through the snowy, rocky ridges and never-ending corridors of pine and spruce trees.

Peacefully absorbed in the beauty of the northern winter wilderness, I began to reflect on my departure from home in southern Ontario four years earlier. I had left as a naïve, excited girl in my early twenties. I now returned an independent woman. From the warm nest of my small town in Baden, and fresh from the greenhouse of Emmanuel Bible College in Kitchener, I landed on the hard, concrete hallways of Winnipeg's high schools. Rather abruptly, I became acquainted with smoking, foul-mouthed teenage city girls in my new work with Campus Life, Youth for Christ. Like butterflies freed from the cocoon, I saw many young lives transformed by encountering the love of Christ. In the process, I too had been transformed.

Now I realized as I drove southward that once again my future looked uncertain. Nevertheless, I was returning to my roots and the familiar scent of Swiss apple pies baking in my mother's oven. Three days of lonely travel ended as I pulled into my parents' driveway. I was home again. At age 25, I had survived on my own and grown like the green plants beside me, but it was still the springtime of my life.

In the autumn of that same year, a tall, taffy-brown-haired man in his mid-twenties also returned to his family roots. Feeling summoned home from Canada's West, Bruce Meyers found himself temporarily settled in the bedroom of his early

Chapter Two

youth, just 15 miles away from my hometown.

He left behind an elementary school classroom in Boise, Idaho where he served as a volunteer teacher's aid for two years. When his mission term ended, he headed north to Calgary, Alberta and revelled in youthful festivities as a camp counsellor for the summer. The years from home cemented his foundation of faith in God and challenged his small world. The building blocks of his life were just beginning to rise and take shape. Home from the west, but unsettled in life choices and careers, we both lacked direction for the future.

In the sphere of relationships, I had slowly resigned myself to living as a single lady. Almost certainly. My ideals for a life companion remained high, causing some painful separations. I desired a mate that shared my calling and dreams. However, discovering a match looked bleak, perhaps impossible.

Through church friends, I soon found employment with the Independent Living Centre, an organization serving people with physical disabilities. To my surprise and delight, this new job would become the crossroads merging the destiny of two lives, an intersection that sparked hopes and dreams.

Within walking distance of work, I settled into an older apartment imbued with charm and character. Morning sunlight poured through the expansive multi-paned windows and nourished my cherished Winnipeg plants in their new setting.

Bruce's name crossed my desk in my downtown office more than once that fall. Staffed in the ILC Apartment Project across the city, he served as an attendant care worker for disabled people. News of his reputation for wild, amusing antics also reached my desk. I had not yet met him but something resonated in my heart just from seeing his name in print. It was a curious thing that I never forgot.

Bruce's demeanour at the formal ILC Christmas banquet appeared reserved and quiet. I felt intrigued. It did not match the reputation of the extrovert I had heard about or seen at a previous party. As an assistant in the organization, I felt it necessary and appropriate to introduce myself to this mysterious fellow worker. I approached him with friendly confidence. Attractively tall and slim, he had huge fawn-like hazel eyes that seemed to peer deeply into my soul. My confidence quickly waned.

It had been only a brief encounter but already I sensed that I overstepped my bounds with this secure man. It struck me odd that he could be so different on two occasions. It struck him odd that I would be so assertive as to introduce myself. *Who was this intriguing man, with such an aura of strength?* I mused. *Who was this bold, independent woman?* He wondered. Later that evening in a staff game of Trivial Pursuit, he further impressed me with his broad scope of knowledge.

The cold winter months passed with no further communication or thoughts of Bruce, until one day at work. I had chirped my usual phone greeting, "Good morning, Independent Living Centre."

"Good morning Marilyn, it's Bruce Meyers from the ILC Project. How are you doing?" My heart skipped a beat when I heard his deep, rich voice over the phone. Gradually his business call evolved into more personal conversation. A friendship slowly began to bud, but my reservations about our differences created a barrier to hopes of anything more serious. I felt drawn to him by his depth and intellect, along with his great capacity for fun. I had also seen his heart for God and his compassion for people. Yet, I held back.

Chapter Two

While settling into city life, I grew increasingly tired of living alone. Feeling certain the rest of the world had companionship and exciting things to do on a Friday evening, I found myself once again forgotten and frustrated. Something needed to change. Riding the elevator to the top floor of the tall, downtown office building where I worked, I headed out to the peaceful garden terrace. In tears of frustration, I cried out to God through the darkness. There I stood, a petite woman calling out from the middle of a bustling city, yet I trusted that somehow He would hear me.

> Lord, please hear my cries. I'm so tired of being alone. I have trusted you for job and finances, my home and material needs, but I have not trusted you to meet my emotional needs. In this I have suffered disappointment. You know that I am willing to go to the mission field, but I am afraid of being left alone on the field, starving for love.
>
> It is time for a soul mate, Lord, the one I can share my life with. I am tired of the pain, the loneliness, and the silly dating game. Please send me a husband. I want to follow you all my life, but I don't want to do it alone.

Wearily returning to my apartment, I journaled the prayer I had voiced toward the starry heavens. It was the first time I made this blatant request of God. Instead I had tested the waters myself far too often and come up empty. It seemed a desperate prayer, far too humbling.

That very evening across the city, Bruce, leaving his work shift felt eager to show someone his newly-purchased touring bike. Biking had become his new passion, offering both transportation and sport. He had little desire to possess a vehicle like most men of his age. Instead he preferred exploring back countryside roads or winding through city alleys. That fall, he planned to cycle the

Rocky Mountains of Alberta and Idaho—a 1000 kilometre trip.

Climbing on his shiny, new, silver touring bike, he began a mental checklist. Which friend would he visit at such a late hour to share in his joy? The lot fell to me.

Sleepy and disoriented, I squinted through the peephole of my apartment door to see who knocked so late at night. An excited, familiar face greeted me from behind a shiny, new bike. Deep into the wee hours of the morning, we conversed and bonded. The evening captivated me, seeming only the beginning of something wonderful. I recorded the joy of that night directly below my prayer in the journal. Over a year passed before I made the connection between the pleading prayer and the timely answer only hours later.

The Princess and the Clown

"No, I will never marry Bruce Meyers!" I announced emphatically in response to teasing by fellow office workers. As our relationship became more public, my resistance towards commitment to Bruce only strengthened. Most certainly he was not the match of my dreams.

In his wisdom my boss, Jim, painted a mental picture of Bruce as a father, "Picture him playing baseball in the fields with his boys—laughing, loving and carrying on. Bruce would be a wonderfully animated, loving and dedicated father," he deliberated. It struck me with its unmistakable truth and opened the door of my heart a crack. I never forgot that poignant image.

As my love for Bruce grew and our daily lives meshed, I needed to address my resistance and our outward differences. To help sort it out, I wrote a poetic piece called *The Princess and The Clown* revealing the contrast in the ways we related to the world. I was a romantic who deemed it necessary to greet the world with dignity and poise. I too, loved adventure and silliness but within limits. He on the other hand presented himself as a free-spirited, nutty character craving laughs and adventures no matter what the social conventions.

For example, one evening we came upon a rusty old shopping cart while walking the streets of downtown Kitchener. He insisted that I climb in. Pushing me wildly down the hilly street, I protested in embarrassment. It was all too much for this young, but mature woman! In his mind, I needed to loosen up a bit.

In our outward appearance, I was considered the refined, classy lady and he, the rugged mountain man who couldn't match two colors together. In our theology, he emphasized the serving expression of the gospel, while my focus had always been evangelism. Could God really be putting these two people together? We seemed as mismatched as his shirts and pants.

In the winter of 1984, Bruce pressed for a commitment. I had reached the wall of decision. Did God want me to climb over it or turn back yet again? Our matters of incompatibility needed to be wrestled with. Slowly God began to show me what was truly needed for a marriage union. The external concerns such as appearance and image would take growth and acceptance, but matters of the soul and spirit were of greater value and importance.

I began to see striking similarities. Our temperaments appeared remarkably similar. Although both extraverted, we also enjoyed quiet intimacy and deep conversation. We shared a love of the arts, literature, music, nature, travel, and people. Most importantly, our dreams and ideals for the future were one. We both desired to live simply, to raise a Christian family, and to care for the poor and lost. Although bearing strongly distinctive identities, we matched as soul mates.

Distant Cries of Africa

We talked of Africa. God sparked the dream in Bruce's heart at a young age. He recounted the memory of a missionary showing slides of Africa at his church. While his eyes focused on the unique images projected onto the screen, the missionary's voice faded as something stirred in his young heart. At age 12, he felt certain he would be in Africa some day.

As the promise of marriage grew, thoughts of Africa became a greater factor in decision making for our future. In the artsy, renowned, town of Stratford, Ontario, we searched for the perfect engagement ring. All the while we kept Africa in mind. The diamond could not be showy and excessive if we planned to be among the poor someday.

Throughout our five-month engagement, many questions began to shape our lives as one. How could we stay in a culture with so much wealth while others around the world had so little? Why had we been given so much? How could we live differently here in Canada so that our lives reflected the message of Christ? These questions would remain in our hearts throughout our married life.

We readily agreed that we could not be content with living a life of mediocre Christianity. Our lives would need to count as passionate followers of Christ. God had long opened our eyes to the needs in the world. In our youth, we each responded to the unconditional love of God and the distant cries of Africa. Now together, we felt certain God had a chosen destiny for us. Someday we would go to the poor.

These were words all so easily spoken, yet so easily forgotten in the whirlwind of life. But God had not forgotten.

Reading books aloud to one another filled our leisure time as newlyweds. One book challenged us like no other. Bruce, unable to receive the depth of its impact on his life, could not bring himself to finish the last chapter. My brother recommended the book *Is that Really You God?* by YWAM founder, Loren Cunningham.

A white ship appeared on the cover. The dream of a ship had been sparked for Don Stephens and Loren while introducing a group of young people to evangelism. Hurricane winds swirling around them while sheltered in an airplane hangar changed the course of their ministry. Devastating effects of Hurricane Hugo in the Bahamas compelled them to respond. There they realized the danger of not expressing one aspect of the gospel: that of loving their neighbour in practical ways. A new concept in missions arose combining evangelism with acts of mercy to reach the world. Using ships as a tool to deliver physical and spiritual aid to the world's forgotten poor, they presented a two-handed expression of the gospel, giving the whole message of Christ.

Total abandonment to our loving heavenly Father and learning to hear His voice plucked deep chords in our hearts as we read the story. We learned how the dream to reach the poor had been cruelly snuffed out when a deal on a ship being prepared for the mission fell through. Many years later that spark of a dream ignited once again when the *Anastasis*—a Greek word meaning resurrection—was purchased. In 1978, a new mission emerged called Mercy Ships.

The story felt personal and real, as though we'd lived it, or were about to. Part of the mystery of our close identification with it could be explained. The concept of two hands expressing the gospel combined the theology and emphasis of our individual upbringing. In joining our beliefs, we readily embraced this whole truth. It was the essence of who we were in our newly married life!

Conviction and destiny surfaced in those early months of married life, but serving the poor from a hospital ship that sailed the world seemed like a lofty, unreachable dream. Perhaps merely the romantic dream of a newlywed couple.

Further education, careers and babies loomed just around the corner. In the next few years we rarely spoke of it again. For a decade, the last chapter of *Is That Really You God?* remained unread. However, the sparks of a dream had been lit in our hearts.

Stage One - The Potter's Wheel

Just a little ball of clay. Then the Lord of life scoops it up with His mighty hand and places it on the Potter's wheel. Gently He begins to shape and mold the new, young Christian. His hands reach into the centre of the clay and we find ourselves spinning, stretching and turning on the wheel. The shape is still a mystery; the destiny is still unknown. If we knew the costly, purifying journey of becoming His chosen, beautiful vessel, perhaps we would try to tear ourselves away from the Potter's wheel.

Joy and child-like trust often characterize the early years in the journey of Christian faith. Like many in their youth, Bruce and I proved idealistic and naïve about the journey of life with the Master Potter. With willing, fearless abandonment to God and to our own ambitions, we made swift decisions about our future. Had we foreseen the troubling years ahead, I wonder how eagerly we would have responded to His gentle hands reaching into the core of our lives.

The Creator would stamp His imprint and destiny into our very being. A unique shape would be molded into the wet, pliable clay. We spun joyfully on the Potter's wheel and He graciously poured out his love. Just when we thought His favour and blessing would last forever, He lifted us off and placed us on the shelf. [1]

3
Tests in the Wilderness

As the clay in the hands of the potter, so are you in my hands, O house of Israel.
Jeremiah 18:6

    Our honeymoon trip to Quebec's Laurentian Mountains drew to a close. Blissfully Bruce and I sat basking in the glorious strains of a live orchestra playing in Montreal's Notre Dame Cathedral. High in the dark, wooden balcony of the old cathedral, Bruce felt the urging of God's Spirit to return to university and finish his education.

    On the final misty morning of our trip, we strolled quietly along a dock in the picturesque Thousand Islands. Bruce stopped and began cautiously sharing his new ambition with me. When we returned home, he intended to enroll as a full-time university student charging me with the sole responsibility of supporting us. I readily agreed, feeling more concerned about putting our lives in order in our new apartment. I thought more about wedding gifts to unpack, thank you notes to write and rooms to organize. It was difficult to look that far ahead when I felt caught up in the thrill of married life and settling into a new role. Besides, I found it a great relief not having to make major life decisions on my own anymore. With the two of us, I felt invincible and securely cushioned from life's pressures.

One month after our honeymoon, Bruce registered for classes at the University of Waterloo. Dissatisfied with my long commute, I resigned from my recent job as a child care worker in Stratford. Thus, our married life began in 1985 with Bruce as a student and me as a newly unemployed housewife searching for work.

Bruce finished his university degree just as I discovered I was newly pregnant. Filled with the joy of expectation, we stood on the threshold of a family and career just before our second anniversary. Together we pursued service in a camping ministry.

As spring rounded the corner, we blindly accepted a position by phone as year-round managers and camp directors in Manitoba. Had we first checked out the camp or earnestly sought God's desires rather than our own, perhaps our decision would have been different. Merrily planning this grand leap of faith, we relied on our own energies along with the naiveté and self-confidence of youth. Later we would stumble in the process.

Scampering squirrels and rabbits greeted us upon arrival at the deserted camp in southern Manitoba. Moist scents of new life emerged through rotted winter debris rendering the air pungent with spring. Taking a much anticipated tour, we observed the condition of the grounds and buildings. Gradually as we toured, it became evident what was truly needed for this camp— maintenance managers. We had been hired primarily for our skills as summer program directors with limited use of Bruce's mainte-nance skills for the year-round winter programs and retreats. Feeling a little concerned, we wondered how this new ministry career would unfold for us.

Situated in Turtle Mountain Park near the International Peace Gardens, miles of wooded hiking trails and fresh lakes surrounded Camp Koinonia. Portaging and canoeing offered children a rustic camping experience. Bruce jumped into the tasks of chopping wood, clearing trails, cleaning the beach front, and purchasing skis for winter rental groups. I set about naming each of the deserted cabins and adding creative touches to the drabness. Updating and organizing files, I created a new camp office. As summer approached, we worked at building strong relationships with the camp board, forging new ground with staff and campers, and making needed changes to the campgrounds.

As our first season wound down and the last car of campers faded into the woods, we revelled in the silence momentarily. While the voices of summer echoed in our minds, we immediately began preparing the camp for winter. Weekend groups would soon arrive for retreats in the snowy park.

That first Manitoba winter, a fierce snowstorm wrapped itself around the camp and isolated me for days. Winds howled angrily at the camp house heaving heavy mounds of snow against it. Roads and pathways disappeared into a white world of oblivion. Bruce phoned to reassure me of his speedy return from a camping conference in Pennsylvania. Heat and electricity became unstable forcing me to devise survival plans. Bundling up our new baby Brandon in a sleigh, I made one attempt in the gusty storm to reach the kitchen of the camp's main lodge. Panting heavily with each step, I tracked through the deep snow that reached up to my thighs. Brandon, sensing the storm around him, howled in his sleigh, increasing my urgency. I had hoped to load up a stash of canned food. But the door of the kitchen, blocked by several feet of snow and frozen stiffly, wouldn't budge. Defeated, I returned in my own deep footsteps. A vulnerable, lonely feeling set in as the days of isolation continued.

After phoning park authorities, I gratefully accepted their offer of ongoing communication and assistance for my stranded baby and me. They assured me that if the storm continued much longer, they would deliver food and baby formula six miles into the woods by snowmobile. To my relief, the electricity returned, the storm subsided and eventually Bruce returned home by snowmobile.

Those days of isolation felt so long and empty. When the storm settled, I stared for hours at the white fur-lined branches from the office window of our camp home. How was it that I found myself so alone in such a harsh, yet beautiful wilderness? The question dominated my feelings during that season of our lives.

Growing times of fellowship in the Whitewater Mennonite church of Boissevain nurtured us like an oasis in the wilderness. These prairie believers excelled at making us feel accepted and welcomed in their community. On weekends, we rode horses through the Turtle Mountain Park trails with some new friends, or enjoyed a meal of watermelon and rollküchen, a traditional Russian Mennonite dish, new to our tastes.

Another unique oasis during that time will always be remembered. Our fourth anniversary fell during the busiest season of summer kid's camp leaving us no opportunity to leave the camp and celebrate. Secretly, the summer staff found a way to honour us on our special day. Dave, the camp cook trained as a chef in a four-star restaurant loved to cook fancy dinners. As their plan hatched behind our backs, Bruce discovered discarded shrimp shells in the sink. Not wanting to embarrass Dave in front of others, he put off confronting him for using the camp's strict budget for elaborate staff snacks. He's glad he did!

That evening, suddenly the staff captured and blindfolded us. Whisked into adjoining canoes, they paddled us out onto Lake Max. The Blue Heron, a pontoon that Bruce had painted and named, anchored motionless out on the lake. Shuttled aboard, staff released the blindfolds and seated us at a small table on the pontoon. Leaving us stranded on the lake, our captors paddled quickly back to camp. We sat in awe of the cuisine set before us. Someone had sneaked into my kitchen and snatched candles, my good china and crystal. A colourful shrimp dish prepared to perfection and a strawberry dessert awaited us. In romantic solitude, we enjoyed our gourmet style supper by candlelight in the middle of the lake. The camp reflected in the distance off the glassy calm waters. Almost a perfect anniversary evening. As dusk settled over the idyllic scene, the happy couple soon became a feast for hoards of blood-sucking insects. The staff had forgotten the mosquito coils! We called for help before we were completely forgotten on the lake. Little did we know that it wouldn't be the last time we shared meals in the middle of a body of water!

In the fall two letters arrived which changed our hearts and set our focus on home. One reached us from Ontario with devastating news. A painful marriage breakdown in Bruce's family shook us deeply. At that time, divorce had rarely touched our homogenous community, let alone our close family. From a distance, we tried to process the news with family members.

The other letter dealt a final crushing blow. An influential summer camp counsellor, whom we'd trusted, had been gently confronted on some issues. He sent a cruel letter venting his resentment towards us. Angrily he scribbled, "Head back to Ontario where you belong!" For me, the sharp arrow hit its targeted mark.

Lonely and hurt, we felt the situation becoming overwhelming. Since our primary skills and gifts were not being utilized effectively, we felt wrongly hired for the job. With each season, the heavy maintenance and camp workload seemed to intensify. Furthermore, I discovered I was pregnant with our second child. Fulfilling my camp role, while raising two babies, increased my anxiety as a new mom. We returned briefly to Ontario with the intent of visiting family and seeking retreat. Walking hand-in-hand through the woods, Bruce and I shared openly and prayed about our future at the camp. Bruce found it much harder to consider leaving despite the pressures and frustrations we faced. He had great hopes for a career in camping ministry. For the sake of his wife and growing family, he made the honourable choice over his own ambitions. Together we asked God for release. The decision was made.

After the blurring months of summer camp ended, we packed all our belongings from our rustic camp home into an old empty yellow school bus. Disappointed and discouraged, we returned to Ontario just a year and a half after leaving. We had been so keen to use our combined gifts and skills as a team in our new married life. Now quickly laid aside, they sat back on the shelf. Failure seemed to have marked us. It was a harsh blow for this newly-married couple.

Now what?

4
Soul Thirst

> *My soul thirsts for you, my body longs for you, in a dry and weary land where there is no water.*
>
> *Psalm 63:1*

Hoping to recover and move on from our disappointing ministry experience, we were unprepared for the distressing event that lay just around the corner.

Finding a semi-detached home in Kitchener, we settled in with our growing family. A sharp contrast to the isolation of the beautiful campgrounds, we felt grateful for the parklands behind our crowded, city home. We awaited the birth of our second child due just 16 months after the arrival of our first.

One evening after settling Brandon into bed, we chatted lightly with Bruce's parents around our kitchen table. While sipping a glass of grapefruit juice, suddenly I felt a warm gush of fluid exit my body. Bewildered, but trying not to appear alarmed, I excused myself discreetly from the table. "Had my water broken?" I chided myself that it was hardly likely at this stage. But the sight of crimson red blood shocked me.

Rushed through emergency, nurses whisked me onto a delivery table. One nurse wished me good luck for my delivery, to which I inwardly responded, "You're crazy, there's no way I'm having a baby yet, I'm only seven months pregnant!"

I had been right about that, but the unnerving bleeding continued intermittently for several days. Doctors now considered me a high-risk pregnancy. I could lose my child. However, my condition returned to normal and doctors released me from the hospital. Anxious to return home to my family, I quickly retrieved a sense of normalcy. Those had been trying days for us all, but if only that had been the end.

Awakened out of a deep sleep, one week later the familiar warm fluid caused me to gasp with fright and waken Bruce. Instinctively, he knew the danger. His face whitened with alarm as he jumped to the emergency!

Again I reluctantly left my toddler son in the hands of grandparents as we raced off to the hospital. Again I found myself lying on a narrow, hard delivery bed hooked up to wires and monitors. Thankfully, the bleeding ceased just like before. However, after extensive tests, poking and prodding, my family doctor broke the news gently, "This time you will remain in the hospital until you have a baby."

"What? ...Are you kidding me? I have a 15-month-old baby at home needing my care!" I protested strongly. "There is no way that I can stay here that long."

Dr. Kennel used a stronger approach, "If you continue to bleed heavily, surgeons have six minutes to perform a C-section before you and your baby's lives are in danger. It's important to keep the

Chapter Four

baby in the womb as long as possible to give it a strong chance of survival. You will likely need a C-section." I finally conceded to his serious tone. With some denial at facing a placenta-previa pregnancy, I made the mental adjustment to separation from my husband and child.

An endless frightening cycle peaked every three to four days. In the quiet darkness of my labour room, the rush of fluid woke me instantly. Nurses responded swiftly to my buzzer. The emergency routine began. Quickly finding a vein, they inserted a needle and started the IV drip in preparation for a threatening C-section. Tightening all my lower body muscles, I made a vain effort to stop the flow. Frightened, I willed and hoped for it all to stop. Willed and hoped that my baby wouldn't enter this world too soon!

Even when my situation settled, I was not permitted to rise out of bed. Life had been put on hold for an impending emergency! Just when my anxiety lowered, light contractions initiated the cycle again. Repeatedly my spirits sank. Each time I descended emotionally, fear gripped me. I felt my life spinning wildly out of control.

After one night's struggle, numerous medical staff surrounded my bed. Stark fluorescent lights shone in my eyes and the strong odour of blood filled the room. My mind created a sense of detachment from my body as it became the property of doctors and nurses. My dignity eroded with each passing day. It all felt totally out of my control. The obstetrician warned me that he would only allow one more hour for the crisis to pass or he would deliver a premature baby. It passed. Relief flooded over everyone. Our unborn child had gained another day in the womb.

Years later while reading a devotional booklet, I discovered why

I met this crisis with considerable struggle instead of trust in God.

> The desire to be in control is one of the strongest drives in the personality. Have you noticed how often when something goes wrong or your life is wrapped in mystery you search desperately for some understanding of why things are the way they are, for then your life seems slightly more under control.
>
> The desire to be in control is one of the greatest enemies of trust...the desire to be in control is not necessarily wrong; it becomes wrong if we use it to provide us with a plan to follow when God invites us just to trust.[1]

I came to realize that I could mentally assent to the fact that God was trustworthy. But under great pressure from the crisis of my pregnancy, my level of trust had revealed itself for what it truly was: trust in myself. Trust in my own ability to control my destiny, to solve my own problems, to be in control of my own body. I never surrendered my pregnant body into the hands of God during that time. Vulnerable and fearful, I fought an inner battle to stay strongly in control…and lost.

The law of opposites also clarified a manner that God used in my life repeatedly over the next few years to grow His character in me. "One of the basic principles of effective Christian living is that whenever God sees a quality that is lacking in us and sets out to develop it, He puts us in a situation where the opposite conditions prevail.

"If God wants to develop patience and perseverance in us then He will make sure we have opportunities to learn how to do so by sending (or allowing us) to have more than our usual share of tribulation. If he wants to develop joy then He will allow us to become involved in circumstances that cause sorrow. If it is peace He wants to develop then we will find ourselves in a situation akin to being in the midst of war. It is the same with trust. To develop trust there is no better way than putting us in a position where we feel we are not in control."[2]

Weak and overcome with self-pity, I had no eyes to see the weariness and battles Bruce faced. In his attempt to keep my spirits raised, he hid them from me. I longed for his visits. He read poetry and Psalms to me, which brought a measure of comfort. It was simply his presence that I desired most.

On the home front, Bruce valiantly prepared meals, kept up with household chores, cared for Brandon's needs, and rushed between baby sitters, work and hospital. Over the years, my husband had proven to be a handyman as well as fully capable in the kitchen and around the home.

Prior to this crisis, Bruce had begun renovations on our small, dingy bathroom. Torn off shower walls exposed old glue and dirty wallboard. The new constraints on his schedule left it in this unsightly condition for weeks. Having also begun a new job in a plastic factory, the stresses and added responsibilities from my absence began to mount up. His body succumbed to a nasty winter flu which overtook him for nearly a week. Returning to the factory with the required doctor's note, he felt shocked to be told he no longer had a job. In disbelief, he quickly requested a meeting with the manager. Appealing on behalf of his short, but good work record, somehow he convinced the manager to allow him to remain.

That evening as he returned home, the pressures seemed insurmountable. Breaking into tears in the ugly, unfinished bathroom, he cried out for strength, "Lord, please don't give us more than we can handle. I'm at the limit." Once he casually commented to me that sometimes he wished he could crawl into the hospital bed and trade places with me. It revealed his struggle.

Through the endless days in my hospital bed, my prayers felt futile. They seemed only to hit the tiled ceiling and bounce back to me as empty, useless words. I stared longingly out the large window of my sterile room wishing my troubles would escape and fly far away into the winter skies. Our new, young pastor visited and prayed for peace in my heart. It seemed beyond my comprehension that I could feel peace at a time like this.

Then a new challenge faced us. Several ultrasound tests were required to ensure that the baby was positioning and developing normally. Oddly, the technician left for a long period of time after the test. Returning, they explained the discovery of a shadow on the baby's brain. "It may or may not be a cause for concern," the obstetrician stated calmly. We chose the latter flatly refusing to accept any more worry.

But deep inside, fear and unbelief seized a broad corner of my heart. I couldn't bear to release the care of my baby and me over to God. Did He really care anyway? I felt no intervention or sense of His presence. Others talked about His amazing presence and comfort during such a time of struggle and anguish. That all seemed like a myth to me now. It certainly wasn't my reality. Fine Christian words that people used for testimonies, but they registered hollow in experience. Perhaps people shared these shallow testimonies out of a sense of duty to God. We must attempt to make our faith seem strong and real, I reasoned. We need to make God look good, even if He doesn't. It all seemed fake and false. Unreal. Discomfort and stressful anxiety about my baby had become my reality of life. As the child grew heavier in my body, the delivery bed felt like a stone slab.

On March 3, 1989, I awoke to the morning sunlight pouring in my room, reflecting a warm rusty red hue off the brass bed. Nurses had moved me to the empty birthing room. My breakfast sat on a tray at the foot of my bed. Just as I reached for it, the frightening warm flow returned. Feeling angry and frustrated, I made a rebellious decision. Refusing to alert nurses, I chose to begin eating my breakfast anyway, and ignored my serious condition. I was a hungry, pregnant lady resentful of being forced into fasting each time this happened.

At that moment Dr. Halmo, my young obstetrician, walked into the room to routinely check on me. Feeling caught with my hands in the cookie jar, I spilled out the truth in tears, "I'm bleeding again and they're going to come in and take away my breakfast and my shower! I had a good day planned and now everything's changed!" I blubbered on in tears. For the first time, this sensitive doctor saw me lose control. He took it as a sign that I'd reached the end of my rope.

"Well, how would you like to have a baby today?" he smiled.

"Really?" I asked in disbelief.

"I think you've had enough of all this. I'll make arrangements for 11:30, but you need to stop eating your breakfast!"

Obediently I shoved it aside and quickly phoned Bruce. I repeated the doctor's words, "Hon, how would you like to have a baby today?"

Chadwick Meyers, born only two weeks premature, weighed in at six pounds, twelve ounces, exceeding the ultrasound prediction of five pounds. Because of the high risk, eight medical people stood present for the delivery. After a cursory examination of our newborn, the pediatrician congratulated us and left. Chad, a healthy baby boy, needed no extra care. Ultrasound revealed that the shadow on his brain had vanished. Bruce's eyes glistened with tears when we received the good news.

Recovery was slow, but knowing I would soon say good-bye to my view of the naked tree-lined streets and snowy rooftops surrounding St. Mary's Hospital brought sheer exhilaration. We had lived with anxiety and gruelling uncertainty for six weeks. I would finally be going home with a new healthy son in my arms! The thought of sleeping in my own soft bed beside my husband felt blissful.

The demands of motherhood gave little time to process the trauma I had lived through. A huge fountain of uncried tears seemed locked inside waiting to be released—tears that were never given the opportunity.

Apart from the sheer delight of our sweet boys and family life, I discovered the adjustment to two babies more stressful than anticipated. Nursing one child, while attempting to potty train the other proved to be a comical recipe for disaster. Bruce and I shared the nightly teething and feeding rounds, waking only for the cry of our designated child. Feeling sorry for myself after an exasperating marathon night I asked him, "Did you know I was up at least four times with Chad last night?"

"No, did you know I was up at least four times with Brandon?" he retorted. Our ears became finely trained to their individual night cries. Sleep deprivation took its toll on our relationship. Silly spats released tension temporarily, but injured the relationship.

Menial tasks of motherhood did little to raise my post partum self-esteem. I sought the luxury of time for myself. The creativity of earlier years deserted me when motherhood marched in the door. Writing poetry or attempting hobbies became a thing of the past. My brain surely had been reduced to the size of an animal cracker. Physically active pursuits left me with aching joints, tiredness and lethargy.

Persistent diapers, feedings, cooking, cleaning, and the reading of thick board books to cuddled-up children filled my days. Sometimes motherhood manifested itself as drudgery, and other days as the pure joy of serving my sweet family. Nevertheless, my role in life had changed, and I keenly felt the heavy yoke of my responsibility.

Quick prayers eked out of a sense of duty replaced long meaningful times spent with God. Although deeply grateful for my son's life, the need for God had been pushed to the deeper recesses of my heart. Buried under the painful weight of Chad's difficult birth and life's more pressing needs, I became oblivious to my spiritual thirst.

5
Silence in the Crib

You turn things upside down, as if the potter were thought to be like the clay! Shall what is formed say to him who formed it, "He did not make me"? Can the pot say of the potter, "He knows nothing"?

Isaiah 29:16

Closely following on the heels of Chad's birthing crisis, tragedy struck near us. Parties and rowdy music of the 18-year-old mother of two often pounded through the walls of our semi-detached home. Her racket had woken us numerous times before, but one morning it sounded different. At the regular 6:30 am baby feeding time, the young woman bounded out of bed and stomped down the hallway. Her heavy steps and shrieks of terror shattered the quietness of the early morning and woke Bruce. Quickly he leaped out of bed. He dressed, ran and pounded on her front door. Her male friend answered. Breathlessly, Bruce informed them that he knew CPR. The door opened instantly.

I listened intently through the wall and prayed for some sign of good news, but instead greater screaming than before followed the moment of silence. Bruce looked at the baby's blue face and the still, silent body in the crib. Turning to her with tenderness, he shook his head and said quietly, "I'm sorry, it's too late."

The distraught mother had given birth just five weeks earlier at the same hospital. In a room down the hall, I'd heard a woman cursing and hollering her way through labour. Nurses complained to me about it. Knowing she was due with her baby soon, I commented humorously that it was probably my neighbour. I had been right. She had given birth to a beautiful daughter.

Now in disbelief, I watched the paramedics carrying her baby away to the ambulance in front of our home. A lifeless limb dangled out of the white blanket. I held my two-week-old son sleeping peacefully in my arms, grateful for his pink skin, grateful that he was alive and breathing. Bruce and I felt desperate to keep holding him all day.

Police arrived to ask questions. Shaken and distraught, we later dressed our children and left our home for the day. The memory of the sweet baby's blue face haunted Bruce. Death had visited under our roof.

The grieving mother only returned once to pack her belongings. Against the red brick home leaned a dismantled crib and orange, floral mattress. April rains wept on that crib. Weeks later, one day it mysteriously vanished. The woman's noisy home had turned deathly quiet.

The incident shook us and raised my vigilance for the whimpers and cries of night-time feedings. Night after night while nursing, I pondered why God chose to take the life of that young infant. *Could this have been His severe mercy to a cruel mother? Why hadn't I made more effort to reach out to her with God's love?* Instead I had griped inwardly about the noise levels and contemplated reporting her to Family and Children services for the bad treatment of her three-year-old son. I had allowed her physical size and fierce mouth to intimidate me and made no effort to connect to her world. In years past I had always reached out in compassion to those around me. I lamented this change.

Outwardly, I seemed an average Christian woman coping with

raising a young family. I knew all the right words, but inwardly they rang hollow. Hence, I said and did little for the cause of Christ. Almost completely unaware, I had made a shift in my spiritual life to the benches of mistrust and disillusionment with God. Since I had always despised hypocrisy, I refused to lower myself to that pew. Being real and authentic were high values in my books. Therefore, silence became my only option.

During those dark nightly feedings, I often attempted to pray. Somehow a heaviness and oppression made praying difficult. Something fearful lurked in that darkness. But I refused to let it affect me, nor did I understand it then.

Instead, my focus and interest in self-help books and secular psychology grew, taking me further away from truth. These books didn't address the truth of my problem—a spiritual one. My view of God had changed in the midst of these times. It is well summed up in this devotional excerpt on giving glory to God.

> ...We think that God is here for our ends and purposes, rather than us being here for his. Modern day Christianity can't receive this too well as it cuts across the present emphasis of: "How can I improve my self-image? How can I be more assertive? How can I solve all my problems?...and so on and so on. We fail to see that God uses fiery trials to get us to focus our eyes on how wonderful and glorious He is.[1]

My spiritual life became an empty, silent wilderness in which I wandered aimlessly. I ignored the thirst and my desperate need to taste the refreshing love and forgiveness of my Heavenly Father. Instead of looking upward, I was looking inward. Unwittingly, I prolonged my own wilderness experience.

Stage Two - The Potter's Shelf

A freshly shaped pot is still soft and incapable of holding water. It requires time on the shelf to dry. This drying, hardening period allows the pot to better withstand the stages ahead without marring or cracking. As moisture escapes, the piece becomes firm, but the smallest knock or shake can cause chipping or breaking.

During this dry season in a Christian's life, there is a sense of abandonment by the Master Potter and an inability to feel His presence or hear His voice. It is like a promotion—but to a spiritual wilderness, where God tests our faith. Will we trust the Potter even when He doesn't seem to answer our prayers? Will we follow with eyes of faith when He eludes us? Will we love and serve Him when the joy is gone and the blessings cease? Are we faithful when we feel spiritually dry and thirsty?

Our camp experience ushered in the spiritual wilderness of our lives. The testing began in the deep disappointment of finding our gifts no longer operative and useful to God. Then God seemed to distance Himself and abandon us at the onset of my troubling pregnancy. But he hadn't. In reality, I'd been given a test to trust Him in the wilderness and failed miserably.

Failing the test of trust, a cool indifference replaced my first love for the Master Potter. Mercifully, the outcome had always rested in God's hands, not my own. And while my soul thirsted and ached, God continued to work out His perfect plan in our lives.

6
Bread of Adversity

Although the Lord gives the bread of adversity and the waters of affliction, your teachers will be hidden no more.
Isaiah 30:19-21

    It was unusual for the phone to ring before breakfast. The call would significantly alter the course of our lives. Newly trained as a cognitive therapist, Bruce left his job in the plastic industrial plant and acquired interesting contract work with brain-injured people. The distressing phone call left him empty-handed. One of Bruce's clients, who'd been making great progress, fell unconscious in a shoe store and died the evening before. The news was a sad blow. Days later another client, subject to poor judgments, dropped his therapy. Administration of the new head injury program moved slowly. Weeks of exasperating unemployment followed as he waited for new contracts. Job security plummeted forcing Bruce to look elsewhere to bring home the bacon.

Stable employment grew into a frustrating venture for Bruce. He'd always believed that his identity and security as a man did not rest in his career. Over the next five years that belief would be deeply challenged. Troubles seemed to tease and lurk around every corner.

Months later, he found a part-time job as a hospital psychiatric attendant. As forewarned, occasionally patients grew violent. Each day he returned home with bizarre stories of strange and repeated crises. The erratic shift work affected our family life, but we felt grateful that it covered the mounting bills. By this time, bringing home the bacon had become more like living on soup! A lifestyle bound by low wages and living on less than the average North American became familiar to us. We groaned under the stretch of our budget and lack of abundance.

Finally, a more secure position as a full-time occupational therapist aide at Freeport Hospital in Kitchener lent stability to our family life. However, the health care field eventually proved unfulfilling and unsatisfying, lacking in a future for Bruce. Something had to change if he was to provide adequately for our family and find long-term meaningful employment.

Wrestling in prayer, he cautiously stepped out in faith and pursued his growing desire to become a teacher. To our surprise, the door flew open through acceptance to teacher's college at the University of Western Ontario for the fall of 1991. The news delighted us and held out the hope of new beginnings for this soup-weary family.

A Sooty Sparrow

The dark, dingy furnace room in our home always bothered me. The door leading to it glowered with a huge black spray-painted swastika sign, left by some previous owner. It always struck me as being weird, along with some of the events that happened there.

Instead of the usual routine before heading off to college, one morning our safe home looked and smelled different. The faint odour of hot rubber changed into a stronger smell like that of a burning motor. Grey smoke began pouring up through the heat registers into each room. Within minutes our house looked like a smoky oven. Coughing and choking, we opened doors and windows gasping for fresh air.

Bruce ran frantically to discover the source of our smoky chamber in the basement furnace room, while I sat helplessly on the living room couch feeling the first stabs of labour pain in my back. Within a few weeks of delivery for our third child, these growing contractions unnerved me. When I informed Bruce of my emerging state on his wild runs about the house, he sloughed me off gruffly and pursued the more pressing emergency. I reacted in a nasty tone causing a brief cross exchange in those moments of crisis. Our coping skills already weakened by life's pressures were slowly being ground down.

He temporarily repaired the problem in the furnace until he had the time to fix it properly. My contractions ceased, proving to be a false alarm as suspected.

However, the disturbances from our grubby furnace room didn't end there. A few days later a strange flapping noise drew our attention to the basement once again. The unfortunate victim, a tiny sparrow, had somehow descended from the skies into the bowels of our home. Reluctantly Bruce slowly opened the latch to the furnace. Dead silence was followed by a rapid flapping of wings as our little prisoner, drawn to the light, escaped above Bruce's head. With a cry of fright, Bruce dashed out of the furnace room cowering into a heap on the floor. I couldn't believe what I was seeing in my husband, until I remembered his story.

Years earlier as a camp counsellor, Bruce had wandered into the woods and unwittingly entered the vicinity of a mother hawk's nest. Angrily she swooped down attacking three times, grazing his head and leaving a part of her talon in his scalp.

Our wee bird was no hawk with a sizeable wingspan, but the sound of flapping wings near his head triggered his past bird encounter. In those few seconds, a sooty little sparrow single-handedly drew out the deep-rooted fear of a grown man. I acted quickly as I watched the male protector of my life crumble. The caged, frightened bird flew wildly about the basement seeking an escape. Isolating it into the furnace room, I closed the door deciding to deal with it later. In the opportune hours during the boys' naps, I made several failed attempts to rid our house of the unwelcome little guest. Finally the next day after Bruce left, I captured the sooty sparrow in a towel underneath the living room sheers. I felt relieved to open the front door and release it to the freedom of blue skies.

The strangeness of those few days stuck with me. The experiences of our smoky home and the sooty bird had tapped into the ugly places of our hearts and brought out the worst. Our cross words to one another, my neediness, and absurd fear resulted in shame for both of us. *Who were we becoming through the ongoing stresses of life?*

Chapter Six

Facing the Mountain

The revelation of a third child in the womb had begun with the same clues—the familiar aversion to lemon detergents and onions. Calculating the arrival date, I had realized I would have three children under the age of three and a half years—just when I was beginning to feel I could cope with motherhood. Routines and toddler independence had made life slightly less demanding and more bearable. Now I faced another mountain.

For several weeks, I resisted the child in my womb as fears took over. The obvious scary question loomed heavily over me. What if this was another placenta previa pregnancy? The unpleasant memories felt fresh—memories I didn't want to repeat. Nausea worsened my gloomy outlook. How I would ever make it through another pregnancy with two toddlers to care for? A new nursing infant meant more night feedings, more teething, more weaning and toilet training. Not to mention the endless hours of washing diapers.

Bruce too, struggled with the news. We agreed that children are a blessing from the Lord, but this one needed better timing! Not only would Bruce be attending college full-time, but we would also face the stress of a baby—another little mouth to feed and no income. Even our pastor jokingly threatened to increase the nursery size if we kept up this pace.

One night after sharing our mutual fears, we held each other while Bruce delivered a heartfelt prayer for strength. He asked God for provision, for a normal pregnancy, for a healthy baby, and for a GIRL! I had a strong sense that God heard us that time.

Regardless of that sense, something wasn't quite right. Unable to peel potatoes for supper while standing, I sat on a stool and lethargically watched each piece curl to the newspaper on the floor. I had hiked a mountain at Lake Louise with reasonable effort during the seventh month of my first pregnancy. Climbing my own stairs now felt far worse than that mountain.

This time the ultra sound showed a properly positioned placenta, relieving my greatest fear. The due date arrived with an otherwise normal pregnancy. Over the months, my love for this unborn child grew and my attitude of dread receded.

Finally the birth day announced itself with sharp pains. Eight hours later, I found myself alone in the delivery room with the lights turned low. I held my peaceful new-born daughter in my arms like a precious jewel from heaven. I spoke softly to her calling her by name. Alert, she searched and fastened her gaze onto my eyes. For a moment, we connected in our spirits and a wee curl of a smile came over her tiny face. Drifting off into infant sleep, it would be days before her alertness matched that window of bonding—a cherished moment that a mother never forgets. Just 20 minutes earlier, my mind, body and spirit knew nothing but fiery pain. The bliss of new life caused me to break into tears of praise to my Heavenly Father. It was the closest I had felt to Him in years.

In answer to our prayers, Jillian, the newest bundle of joy graced our home and filled us with delight. The boys hovered continuously over her pine cradle in the living room. Friends and family, overjoyed with the news of a baby girl, showered our home in shades of pink. Flowers, lacy outfits, gifts and blankets of pink draped everywhere. Not a care in the world, Jillian slept angelically in her pink gingham dress—the one her daddy purchased for the homecoming. Perhaps life with three little ones would be manageable after all.

7
Beauty from Ashes

I will thoroughly purge away your dross and remove all your impurities.
                                          Isaiah 1:25

    I longed for my husband's presence during his long day of commuting to and from London, Ontario. Bruce ventured into teacher's college with renewed enthusiasm, while I spent my days alone with three young ones. Upon his return, I reported all the sweetness and silliness of his young brood, prior to his retreating to a corner for homework.

One incident stands out in my collection of toddler stories. While breastfeeding Jillian one morning, Chad, then two years old, watched curiously. Inquiring innocently he pointed to my right breast, "Milk, mommy?"

"Yes, Chad," I replied.

The wheels were turning in that young analytical brain of his when he pointed to my left breast and asked, "Juice, mommy?"

I held in my laughter with this mental picture of myself as the milk and juice dispenser mom. "Line up, kids. Milk on one side, juice on the other!" Some days, I felt like a dispenser!

The boys' hero dad romped and wrestled every evening after supper on the living room floor. Bruce modelled fun and laughter through the simple things, like games and play-acting. In their eyes, Mom gave them food, but dad gave them fun!

In the pleasures of our family life, my joy slowly dampened with a new growing fear. During private moments, I began to conceive the possibility that I was dying. I grew more disconcerted when strange symptoms manifested themselves in my weary body.

Why was my hair falling out and my voice sounding raspy? Why were rashes appearing on my body? Why was I suffering a strange dizzy feeling? It all confused me. One day while carrying Chad, dizziness threw me off balance and I tripped down the carpeted steps. Holding him upright and safe, my body crumpled underneath me in pain. I gripped the rail strongly to keep from tumbling further. What was happening to me?

I once delighted in surprising people with my muscle strength despite my small size. My growing weakness showed up peculiarly in the simplest tasks. Sugar bowls and jars of jam dropped out of my hand and a basket of laundry toppled to the floor.

My heart thumped heavily and slowly. Breathing became

short and sluggish as though a heavy anvil laid on my chest—a weight weakening my life. Daily my energy level faltered and plummeted. The weariness became indescribable, but my doctor's response to my profound fatigue was predictable. What did I expect caring for three pre-schoolers while breastfeeding?

On a grey November day, Bruce arrived home to find supper unmade. Instead I lay on the floor with my head under the rocking chair while the kids happily played around me. He bent over me with concern in his eyes. "I can't cope," was all I managed to say.

Normally with the dawn of each new day, my disposition had always been sunny and vivacious. I grew more and more perplexed with the change. Feeling bleak and lethargic, some mornings my body would not rouse. I forced myself to crawl on hands and knees to the bathroom. Mild depression hung over me like a heavy cloud.

Then, what seemed an unusual coincidence can only be seen as divine intervention. Chad's pediatrician spotted a mild goitre on my neck. Results of blood tests brought a quick diagnosis of severe hypothyroidism. The diagnosis explained numerous unanswered questions in my life, while medication and life-long treatment brought the hope of stability. I felt thankful it was not a major disease, but it had certainly been wreaking havoc in my life for several years.

For nine months Red Cross Homemakers lent their services to this recovering mother of three. They tidied our home, washed and folded our clothes, scrubbed the floors and played with the children while I rested. I found it intrusive to have strangers doing my housework, but my choices were limited if I was to conserve energy for nurturing my young children.

Home-made soups became the common fare in our household once again during that year of teacher's college with no income. God's provision also came through church friends, parents and our own small garden. A Christmas hamper with food and gifts appeared at our door while a car roared away mysteriously into the dark night.

Keenly ready for a change from our difficult way of life, we celebrated with joy when Bruce finished the year at teacher's college. Wearing his graduation cap and gown, he raised his diploma high in the air. We set our sights high on the hopes and dreams ahead—good health, a growing family, material blessings and a school classroom that Bruce could call his own.

Roots en Route

Our new plan emerged quickly. We put our semi-detached home up for sale and felt pleased when it sold the first weekend on the market. It held five years of sweet memories and hard struggle. Within five weeks we'd found a new home in Seaforth, a small town in rural Ontario. I loved the beautiful image and sound of that name. As the name indicates, it is situated 20 minutes from Lake Huron, one of Ontario's Great Lakes. Having been landlocked most of our lives, this new location delighted us.

We placed ourselves strategically near three counties in south western Ontario. Occasions for supply teaching would be greater, raising the opportunity for full-time employment in the future. Our strategy failed miserably. In the year of 1992, Ontario teachers faced an economic crisis. Cutbacks, budget slashes and hiring freezes became the order of the day. And then the order of the years.

Once again, the quest for employment found Bruce practicing

Chapter Seven

cognitive therapy along with occasional supply teaching. As clients recovered through therapy following their brain injuries, their needs declined. Bruce constantly worked himself out of a job. School principals, pleased with his teaching, longed to offer him a position but the political scene tied their hands. Our hands felt tied by our financial woes.

Then to my chagrin, returning to normal health was not quite the ease I had expected. Doctors had no answers. Striving for wellness felt like chasing a dangling carrot always outside my grasp. Life had changed since the birth of my third child. My high-energy personality felt trapped inside a low energy body. Being highly productive had always brought me great fulfillment in life. Feeling a sense of dismal loss, I now lived with an energy limitation that frustrated me. Pushing those limits only left me fatigued again and again. The most painful realization was that my children would grow up never receiving the best of my youthful vigour. Living with an invisible disability, the quality of our lives had changed.

Feeling robbed and angry, I chose not to roll over and accept this new existence. I researched thyroid disease till I grew weary of seeing it in print. No answers emerged.

As the days passed, I slowly became desperate for God to intervene. With every ounce of spiritual strength I possessed, I trusted the Great Healer to touch and restore my body to its former self. Instead, I felt jarred by a new revelation. On my quest through Christian books and teaching on healing, I was about to find a purpose for my fiery trials.

Oswald Chambers expressed the shift I had made earlier in my spiritual life while sitting through the dry shelf years.

> Is your mind focused on the face of an idol? Is the idol yourself? Is it your work? Is it your idea of what a servant should be...? If so, then your ability to see God is blinded. You will be powerless when faced with difficulties and will be forced to endure in darkness. If your power to see has been blinded don't look back on your own experiences, but look to God. It is God you need. Go beyond yourself and away from the faces of your idols and away from everything else that has been blinding your thinking. Wake up and accept the ridicule that Isaiah gave to his people, and deliberately turn your thoughts and your eyes to God.[1]

How long had I been blinded by my own thinking? I shuddered. Some time in the prior few years, I had yielded to myself and turned my eyes away from God. I had fallen to the philosophy of this age to look within one's self. A pampering in the name of self-worth. My personal journaling revealed a shameful preoccupation with my ego, the need for approval and recognition and motives tainted by self-glory.

As the scales from my spiritual eyes fell away, I examined my heart. The illumination felt unpleasant and deeply disappointing to me. It grew ugly and disgusting to look at. Deep inside me, ugly roots had grown while en route through the spiritual wilderness. Roots of criticism, selfishness, pride and anger needed to be pulled from the soil of unbelief in my life. Humbled before God, I realized I could not request healing for my body while my heart remained sick with the disease of sin and self-absorption. Instead I needed serious heart cleansing.

I now had a choice to make. I could choose to be refined by the fires in my life or refuse their work and find them burning on in vain. It hardly seemed a choice. Pointless suffering or beauty from the ashes.

Chapter Seven

In deep repentance over the next several months, I slowly turned away from the idol of self. I asked God to tackle the root of anger first. Having grown up a compliant child, anger had never been a familiar emotion. In recent years, it became a venting source all too frequently. My frustrations sought a place to blame and vent; yet it never felt right to point the finger at God. Like Eve of old, the finger pointed towards my husband—the reason for all our troubles. I resented him for the instability, for the survival mode we found ourselves in, and his inability to nurture me properly during these difficult times. Although I never voiced this quite openly, the messages were clearly received.

I had set foot on a dangerous path—a path of destruction that could leave a wake of disaster. The strain on our marriage led to painful conflicts that left us both licking our wounds. In my anger, I had become a vicious fighter with words. Oh, the power of that little tongue!

I knew that expressing unrestrained anger damaged others, and that anger left burning internally damaged myself. Feeling confused about this, I began searching for answers from the right source. What did scripture exhort me to do with my anger and unforgiveness? Quite simply, I discovered it commanded, *"Put it away. Repent of it, get rid of it. Forgive."* And so I did. The Holy Spirit did the rest over time. I also confessed my anger to Bruce. He graciously forgave.

While vacationing at the lake that summer, I shared my inner journey with Bruce. Eventually it led to revealing my deepest fear about our relationship—that of outdistancing him spiritually. It stemmed from my fear of us growing apart, but instead it had created a wider gap. I relayed how that led me to compromise my intimacy with Jesus for so many years.

Bruce encouraged me to grow, to soar, and to be all God wanted me to be. This response surprised me. Obviously he felt secure enough to allow me to flourish in my own walk with Jesus. Inwardly, he rejoiced because it released him from the heavy chains of expectation and allowed him to grow at the pace God intended.

Clearly I saw how in my desire for emotional intimacy, I had put things backwards. For years, I'd poured more energy into my marriage than my relationship with Christ. I'd handed the responsibility for my spiritual growth over to Bruce and then blamed him for my lack of growth. A radical shift was needed to put Jesus first. Changing my familiar approach felt akin to jumping off a cliff. To let go and dare to draw nearer to Christ offered no guarantee of a closer marriage. Yet to place my dependency for spiritual growth on my mate rather than on Christ Himself carried a greater risk.

The change in our marriage became dramatic. I fell in love with my husband all over again. In our ninth year, it felt renewed like springtime. Freshly released, Bruce grew leaps and bounds in his spiritual walk. Together, yet separately, we grew.

The critical spirit, weakened by the loss of my anger, slowly faded. The world around me began to look different. With new eyes, I appreciated people instead of inwardly dwelling on their faults. I recognized that because I felt wretched about myself for so long, I had consoled myself by criticizing the weaknesses of others.

Surrendered again to God's powerful love, I felt like a child. God had been resisting my pride all along and would again extend grace to me. From then on, I made a vow to keep my life in strict alignment with God's Word and never wander foolishly again.

Wonderful changes in our life and marriage filtered through

to our young family. That Easter, our children each wrote a personal sin on a piece of white paper. Young Jill needed help to write "hitting my brothers" on her slip. Each one took turns nailing their paper to a crude cross made with branches from our yard. On resurrection Sunday, Bruce quietly disposed of the papers. When the children awoke, the sins had mysteriously vanished! Together we celebrated this poignant picture of forgiveness.

Stage Three – The Potter's Kiln

The clay piece has shrunk slightly during the long drying process on the shelf. Gently removed, it is ready to be placed in the kiln. Temperatures in the kiln are lower at this stage since only a half firing is needed to allow the application of the glaze at a later stage. In the heat of the first firing, all the impurities in the clay start to melt away.

By the hand of the Master Potter, the heat turns up in our lives. As the first fires grow, the Lord starts shutting all the doors and windows, and the fire comes through the floor and ceiling. Our attention turns upward and we feel our need for God to intervene. We cry out, "Lord, are you there?"

Anger, resentment, bitterness and greed all rise to the surface in the midst of the flames. When the fires move from bright red to blazing orange, our best relationships become strained or finances are cut off. We cry out, "Lord! If you love me You'll turn off the heat!" As the sweat starts to drip, we look at the people next to us and decide we don't like them. Sometimes the heat engulfs whole families and churches, exposing the impurities of many hearts all at once.

As the Potter's refining fire touched our lives and marriage, little by little, this impure vessel was transformed. Sludge and impurities burned off, my cool indifference melted and I returned humbly to the Master Potter. The joy of my first love was restored! And for a time, the flames ceased.

8
Currier & Ives

He who dwells in the shelter of the Most High will rest in the shadow of the Almighty.

Psalm 91:1

    Snow drifted to the earth like light white cotton balls. The setting looked like a calendar picture for Christmas Eve. Our quaint country church was only a short walk down the street from our home. Cedar garlands and red bows decorated the old church's wainscoted walls while flickering candles lit the window ledges. The familiar musty church scent blended with the pleasant aroma of the tiny flames, the fresh cut evergreens and women's perfumes.

In the dimly lit sanctuary, people filed into the pews in reverently subdued excitement. On the old upright piano, I began softly playing the prelude—*O Holy Night*. A memorable and meaningful Christmas Eve service followed. As our happy, young family walked home holding mittened hands, the yellow glow of the street lights revealed the steadily thickening blanket of snow. It felt so peaceful and tranquil on this holy night. I reflected longingly on the scene of the birth of our Saviour centuries earlier. Indeed in this corner of the earth, all was right with the world.

Life settled into a pleasant routine in our small town setting of Seaforth. Welcoming stability, Bruce and I purposed to put down deep roots. We endeavoured to walk quietly in submission and humility before God and our neighbours. We deeply cherished our friends and growing children. Weekly teaching and caring support from our pastor restored us from our former troubles. The fellowship at our growing country church grew satisfying and sweet. This peaceful season is exactly how I had imagined life as portrayed by Currier & Ives in paintings years ago. If only life could remain like this forever.

Stage Four – Unglazed Pot

The heavy door of the kiln opens and the clay vessel is removed. The pot has been fired, but is still not glazed. Its overall appearance has only changed slightly, but to the touch the vessel feels different—more durable and less fragile. Water can't be poured into an unglazed pot, because it will leak. Nor can grain be stored in it, because bugs can get inside. The only use for the unglazed pot is to be set back on the shelf to cool.

Relieved to be out of the hot fires and back on the shelf, as Christians we sit quietly in the pew. By now we understand that God is a holy, dangerous God who will stop at nothing to accomplish His purposes in our lives. We've been through the fires, we've paid our dues. Now we become pew sitters and perfect the art of sitting in the shadows of the church.

Awakened by Tall Ships

Visits as a family to marinas and beaches on Lake Huron became more frequent. A vast body of blue, diamond-sparkling waters soothed our spirits and brought solace and peace. Drawn like a magnet, we soaked in the view of distant horizons and ceaseless waves lapping the shore. Barefoot and wearing a flowing white sailor dress, I loved to walk hand-in-hand with Bruce on the beach. Towards sunset hours, while our rosy-faced children happily created creatures and sand castles, I often strolled in solitude pouring out my heart to God, the Lover of my soul.

One warm June day while examining the yachts at a marina near St. Christopher's Beach in Goderich, we discovered a wooden sailing ship—a smaller replica of the tall ships. The entire family ran to get a closer look. Fascinated by the creaking of the mooring ropes, the shiny wood, and the thought of sailing on this vessel, I became aware of something new awakening in my spirit. Ships had never held any fascination for me before this day. The distant memory of a dream surfaced momentarily in my mind.

Remember the dream? The dream of sailing to the poor…

A slight discontentment with our settled, comfortable lives began to emerge and drew me towards God. I sensed Him calling me to a deeper walk and a greater destiny. By now, I had read Jill Austin's article called *In the Hands of the Master Potter*. It spoke of the price for being willing to follow Christ in full surrender. The article impacted me deeply as I looked back at the journey of our lives.

This beautiful potter and clay allegory from scripture seemed to describe our own journey with God. I began to understand that the fires of struggle we'd walked through actually evidenced His great love and discipline, not His displeasure. From youth, I had always strained to believe I was worth loving, but in actuality, God was showing me how much He loved me. Throughout my life His loving hand remained profoundly evident. This had been particularly hard to grasp while prayers remained unanswered and troubles battled against us.

My deeper question remained. *Why was a loving God causing us to suffer?* Oh, the question of the ages! It persists as a dangerous tool in the hands of the enemy to keep us from God! How easy it is to doubt His love by looking at unexplained circumstances. The enemy loves for us to embrace these doubts. It wreaks havoc in our spiritual lives and leaves us groping in defeat. "The essence of Christian faith is to believe God despite 'the evidence of our lying eyes,' for 'we walk by faith, not by sight.' If God is not good, if the suffering of this world is not justified in some way beyond our ken [knowledge], then Christianity falls like a house of cards."[1]

I began to realize that primarily we suffered because of what it would build in our lives and character. For Bruce and me, the trials slowly forced us out of self-reliance and taught us to rely on Jesus, as in the case of my illness. But just like a leaky pot in the unglazed stage, this new knowledge and understanding would be challenged again and again in the higher fires throughout our lives.

The new stirring—this calling to a greater place of intimacy with the Master—needed forethought and consideration. *What would the Master require?* Caution replaced the naiveté of early years as we matured and counted the cost. Total abandonment to God could possibly mean more fire in our lives, more pain and more sacrifice. Were we prepared to pay the price? Surely we had had enough, I assured myself.

To ignore the stirring of God and allow myself to grow

increasingly distant from Him would take me back to the wilderness years, which I had vowed never to return to. Yet to rest at this stage (cooling on the shelf) would only mean stagnation and little growth. Talents and gifts wasted, character unchallenged. Refusing to move onward would keep us in a position of mediocre Christianity and lukewarmness, something we had agreed before God in our early-married life never to fall into. To ignore God's wooing meant shunning the Lover of my soul. It became clear that Bruce and I could no longer stay in this comfortable season. At first, as we cautiously yielded, His plan whispered ever so quietly.

Stage Five - The Potter's Glaze

Slowly, the Master Potter carries the unglazed pot off the shelf to a room full of tables in preparation for the glazing.

At this stage, something deep inside the Christian begins to stir. It's the sense of destiny felt as a new believer. We say, "Lord, I don't want to stay in the back row and die! You made me to be a lover of your people—to find broken vessels and bring them into the Potter's house."

"There's a soft sound of weeping as vessels that have been together all their lives are separated. God is starting to prepare His vessels to fulfil His great commission. Some will be staying home, but some will be travelling to foreign lands.

The angels carefully brush the glaze onto each vessel before carrying them into a large kiln." [2]

9
Embers of a Dream

Then I heard the voice of the Lord saying, "Whom shall I send? And who will go for us?" And I said, "Here am I. Send me!"
Isaiah 6:8

An intense new desire stirred in my heart—a quest to hear the voice of God. Scripture says that His sheep hear His voice and know Him (John 10:27). If this was truly the case, I needed to know for certain that I was hearing His voice. My spirit began to listen for those whispers of the inner voice in my daily time spent with God.

I understood from scripture that we hear voices: the voice of self (our own understanding), the voices of others (friends), the voices of the powers of darkness (Satan), and the voice of the

Chapter Nine

Shepherd (His Holy Spirit). Learning to distinguish these voices and know the Shepherd's became my new goal. Becoming more receptive to God's Spirit followed more naturally for me when surrounded by the beauty of creation. Thus my daily practice of holding my quiet devotional time by a window or out of doors became habitually ingrained.

In my new quest, I returned to the book *Is that Really You God?* read ten years earlier. There, in the summary, I discovered important principles for hearing God's voice—His personal revelation to me.[1]

First, I needed to ask God to help silence my own thoughts, desires, and the opinions of others. Dying to my own imaginations was necessary in order to seek the mind of God (Prov. 3:5, 6; II Cor. 10:5). Second, since the enemy tries to deceive me, I needed to resist Him by using the authority which Jesus gives to silence Him (Eph. 6:10–20; James 4:7). A former fear of demonic activity had fallen away as I grew in faith and understanding of my authority in Christ. Third, I needed to be sure my heart was clean by confessing any unforgiven sin (Ps. 66:18; 139:23-24). Fourth, following the heart check, I was in a position to ask the Holy Spirit to speak His truth to me (Rom. 8:26, 27; Eph. 5:18). I learned to patiently wait in silent expectancy for the Father to speak (Ps. 25:14; Ps. 62:5; 81:13; Micah 7:7).

I discovered that waiting and listening is not an easy part of prayer. If I hear nothing I often grow impatient and allow my mind to wander off or to seek my own voice. Self can be a huge block in being open to the Spirit's voice. There will be times when God is silent; it truly is a miraculous privilege to have personal communion with the God of heaven. In this I'm aware that I've moved past faith as an intellectual exercise and belief, to intimacy with God. I believe this is what it means to truly know Him.

> I know my sheep and my sheep know me - just as the Father knows me and I know the Father.
>
> John 10:14

As I listened for the shepherd daily, the adventure grew. At times God simply gave me one word that whispered into my spirit. That one word could offer comfort, direction or confirmation. Other times a scripture reference came to me and I eagerly looked it up to find it suited my circumstance. Like manna dropped from heaven, it fed my spirit. On more rare occasions, God gave a picture in my mind which seemed a mystery, but later circumstances brought clarity or fulfillment. And I knew that I knew that God had spoken!

My heart being open and ready, I felt stirred whenever I read scriptures relating to the poor. The parable of the rich fool in Luke leapt off the page.

> Then he said, 'This is what I'll do. I will tear down my barns and build bigger ones, and there I will store all my grain and my goods. And I'll say to myself, "You have plenty of good things laid up for many years. Take life easy; eat, drink and be merry. But God said to him, 'You fool! This very night your life will be demanded from you. Then who will get what you have prepared for yourself? This is how it will be with anyone who stores up things for himself but is not rich toward God.
>
> Luke 12:18-21

It struck me that in this wealthy country, we are like the rich fool described in this scripture. *Were Bruce and I too busy struggling to store up goods here on earth?* So far, our focus seemed more like survival. *But were we living our lives only for ourselves?*

And how can we be **rich towards God**? Storing up heavenly

Chapter Nine

treasure seemed to be linked with giving up what we cling to and giving to the poor. Then how is it that vast numbers of Christians ignore these verses, including us?

> From everyone who has been given much, much will be demanded; and from the one who has been entrusted with much, much more will be asked.
>
> Luke 1:48

As I considered our lives, I concluded that Bruce and I had indeed been entrusted with much. We'd been given much by our North American blessings, taught much through our education and diverse churches, equipped much through our combined gifts, and prepared much by our difficult journey. Yet, were we really ready to make a major life change at this stage? Maybe someday, but surely not now.

> No one who has left home or wife or brothers or parents or children for the sake of the kingdom of God will fail to receive many times as much in this age, and in the age to come, eternal life.
>
> Luke 18:29

This verse proved the most disturbing of all. Was God asking us to leave our home, our family and friends? Surely, this would come at too great a cost! I needed to be concerned for our children, I reasoned. To break their strong attachment to grandparents and cousins would shake their young world. Our community of believers around Seaforth had become too valuable to give up. Besides, would God ask us to leave in the midst of strong church growth when our roles seemed vital? Bruce had been recently appointed as an elder, chairman of the board and Sunday school teacher, while I served as worship leader. Furthermore, it made no sense to raise our children in a poor country when our own country had far more to offer them.

Compelling, disturbing and imploring, His voice in scripture became difficult to ignore. But a growing desire to respond churned into a frustrated longing to make a difference in this needy world. *How could I ever fulfill this from my kitchen, and from the constraints of my comfortable home?*

While attending to my duties as mother and homemaker, for months the Master's voice echoed in faraway places of my mind.

Remember the dream.

Ten years had passed since the sparking of a dream God had placed in our hearts. Only dying embers of the dream remained —that of sailing on a hospital ship offering hope and healing to the poor.

As I seriously considered the possibility of missions, I rationalized that I didn't possess the apostle/missionary gifting, nor the fortitude needed to cross cultures. I enjoyed the comforts and conveniences of a microwave, a blow dryer and all the privileges of a North American lifestyle.

Then I reasoned with God. If He were truly sending us to the poor, then He would have to make that clear to my husband too. As confirmation, I asked God to speak to Bruce without my intervention. That would definitely buy me some time. I left it with God feeling quite certain it would be years before anything would surface.

Only three months passed before Bruce approached me with the possibility of going into missions. His leading from God had been remarkably parallel to my leading. Yet Bruce hesitated to say anything for fear that I wasn't ready to hear. The discovery of God's separate leading confirmed His special purpose for our lives.

The embers of the dream ignited once again. God had been blowing on them for years!

Chapter Nine

Eagerly I requested information from various mission organizations, inquiring about the need for teachers overseas. Hearing that teachers were always in demand on the mission field, it seemed unusual that Youth with A Mission and Mercy Ships were the only organizations to respond immediately with the need. Surely this confirmed our dream!

Moving forward, we applied to Mercy Ships International for the required training needed to become long-term crewmembers. Confidential reference forms filled out by several people needed to be mailed back and gathered. Finally we stapled it all together and tucked it in an envelope bound for Texas.

To our dismay, a letter returned apologizing for sending the incorrect application form. We'd filled out an associate crew (short-term) form. The entire process needed to be repeated on a long-term crew form. After all that work, a deep sigh of disappointment was all we could express to one another.

This response to our first attempt at pursuing our dream of missions became a convenient excuse not to continue in our courageous pursuit. Despite what we considered God's leading, we still felt unsure and fearful. If the dream really was God-given, he would bring it to pass in His timing.

In Oswald Chamber's devotional book, his words also encouraged us.

> When God gives you a vision and darkness follows, wait. God will bring the vision He has given you to reality in your life if you will wait on His timing. Never try to help God fulfill His word. Abram went through thirteen years of silence, but in those years all of his self-sufficiency was destroyed. He grew past the point of relying on his common sense. Those years of silence were a time of discipline, not a period of God's displeasure. Isaiah 50:10 -11[2]

The door to serving with Mercy Ships had not completely closed, but it seemed to be one not easily opened. So we simply waited. Gradually overshadowed by life and its demands, the fanned embers of the dream flickered and faded once again.

10
Smoky Kiln

> *Who then devised the torment? Love.*
> *Love is the unfamiliar Name*
> *Behind the hands that wove*
> *The intolerable shirt of flame*
> *Which human power cannot remove.*
> *We only live, only suspire*
> *Consumed by either fire or fire.*
>   T.S. Elliot - *Little Gidding*

Our home seemed too small. We needed more space. As our children's bodies stretched and grew, it felt like we'd outgrown our home like a baby outgrows its crib. Jasmine, our new orange tabby cat joined us on Jillian's fourth birthday. A yearning to own a home in the country emerged. We dreamed of teens enjoying the freedom to ride horses, own pets, and host youth barbecues.

Nestled in the sprawling farmlands of Huron County, down a long tree-lined lane sat a century old farmhouse with a typical Ontario bank barn. Crawling up the rafters onto the straw bales,

I envisioned my children spending long enjoyable hours in the barn as I had done at my grandfather's farm during the summer. As we toured the grounds and the old home, my elation grew over the possibility of declaring this place home for our family. The price was better than right!

That hopeful morning of our final tour with the realtor, I had received a verse from God giving certain direction. It read: *"Instead of the thorn bush will grow the pine tree, and instead of the briers the myrtle will grow."* (Isaiah 55:13) In my excitement I looked up myrtle in my book of plants and trees. I discovered that myrtle doesn't grow in Canada, but that a domestic version called periwinkle does. Ah, there must be pines and periwinkle growing on the property as confirmation from God! To our disappointment, we found only a huge grove of tiger lilies, thorn bushes and spruce trees. I tried to ignore the silly verse. Later, as Bruce and I prayed for God's will on the matter, he voiced what I already knew God was saying, but didn't want to accept. We were not to buy that home.

In angry tears of disappointment, I sought understanding from God. "Why do you choose not to bless us? Why do others seem to receive the desires of their heart, but not us?" I murmured. We let the house go; knowing the opportunity of ever finding another for such a price was remote.

It was only one of a series of disappointments. Knocking on several new doors for employment, one by one each closed painfully. Bruce lost an opportune teaching position in a prison because of wrong certification. After coming home with the disappointing news, he mowed the lawn furiously while I searched the scripture in tears. God opened my eyes to a verse that I would ponder in my heart for a long time.

Chapter Ten

> ...You will weep no more. How gracious he will be when you cry for help! As soon as he hears you, he will answer you. Although the Lord gives the *bread of adversity* and the *waters of affliction,* your teachers will be hidden no more. With your own eyes you will see them. Whether you turn to the right or the left, your ears will hear a voice behind you saying, This is the way, walk in it.
>
> Isaiah 30:19 - 21 (emphasis added)

Bread of adversity and waters of affliction had often been our diet throughout the years. We knew there had to be more from God than simply bread and water.

For two years, Bruce slugged away in a steel factory in Stratford. Sweating it out, he lifted up to 25 tons of steel a day. Two separate hernia operations resulted for him from the lifting. Teasingly, I commented that I'd married a man with brains, not brawn.

As promise of jobs echoed in the news and among teachers, he made another attempt to re-enter the field of education. While hanging on to the security of his factory pay cheque, supply teaching increased, often making it necessary to work the two jobs in a day. Driving immediately from a full day of school, like Superman he changed costumes and roles to begin the three to eleven shift at the steel factory. Rising early in the morning before his family and then retiring after all were bedded down; we passed like ships in the night. To ensure continued communication and strong family life, for several months I kept a family journal to record the daily happenings and messages. During his early breakfast, he responded with letters in the journal. The children painstakingly wrote notes to their father in the family journal. One night Brandon began to cry as he changed into his pajamas. "When is Daddy going to quit the factory job? We never get to see him." I rubbed his back while my heart ached for him. Bruce's notes to me supported me through another long, lonely day.

> Let your love shine through to the children tonight while I work yet another night in the drudgery of evenings alone. Remember the Saviour. Remember our salvation. I love you.
> - Bruce

Finally, he ended the factory days when a foreman pressured him about arriving late from having two jobs. That fall, along with the autumn leaves, Bruce's hopes of ever teaching fell to the ground. Misty-eyed, together we watched as our youngest child boarded the school bus. All curls, bounce and eagerness, she climbed aboard. It was Jillian's first day of kindergarten—a milestone that ended cherished, but exhausting, pre-school years. As the bus roared out of sight, Bruce and I turned back into the empty house. All was quiet. The reality of unemployment set in with its despairing grip. Another school year, four years since teacher's college, and still Bruce had no classroom to call his own.

At age 37, the death of his career dream and years of accumulated struggle seemed beyond Bruce's ability to endure. Depressed and feeling unable to cope, I watched him fall prey to the lies of the enemy. One day in tears of agony, he declared himself a failure as a father and provider. As his caring wife, I resisted this declaration as best that I could, but my words fell empty on the wounded depths of a broken heart. The man I had first been attracted to for his inner strength had been crushed by life. Broken by God. I felt helpless. I knew that only God could put the pieces back together again.

Chapter Ten

Bare Cupboards

Mother Hubbard's rhyme seemed to mock me. "When she got there, her cupboards were bare and then her poor [children] had none." We needed groceries badly. Cringing all the way, I drove slowly downtown and with my eyes fixed on the ground, I walked straight toward the Seaforth Food Bank. To my humiliation, a lady from our church worked behind the counter that day. With eyes of compassion, she handed me bags of food. I drove home in tears of frustration and shame. As financial pressures squeezed and constricted, it became my weekly routine.

Time marched on in this world and we felt left behind. While friends and peers merrily continued to heap assets and settle strongly into careers, for us the situation seemed reversed. All our expectations for success and stability as we approached our 40's lay like a wilted unopened rosebud.

Unspoken doubts of God's love harassed me. Raw, painful questions nagged like some irksome pest I couldn't wave away. *Why did God seem to bless and care about others, but not us? Was there something wrong with us? Were we disobedient? Why must we struggle at every turn? Maybe we didn't deserve His favour in our lives.*

Feeling deeply distressed and desperate for help, we visited Bruce's Aunt Eleanor and Uncle Ray, the pastor who had delivered the sermon at our wedding. Thick, grey fog enveloped our car as we travelled to their home. In those few brief hours, as we shared our struggle and sought counsel, we felt loved. But we felt beyond comforting. We had lost hope.

A black nothingness like the fog seemed to surround us as we returned home that dark night. We had nothing left. No dreams. No future. No money. No energy to knock on any new doors.

We'd reached the end of ourselves—like a slow death inside a smoky kiln.

Remember the Dream

Besides the joy of our children, a persistent impression kept us persevering through the bleakness of those tough winter months. Remember the dream—the call to make a difference in this world.

The faint, distant voice of the Master's plan echoed through the despair and once again it offered us a glimmer of hope. Two years had passed since we first applied to Mercy Ships. The timing had not been right but God had not closed the doors; He had simply asked us to wait.

A new picture persistently entered my mind. A tropical paradise beach, lush spring green palm trees and misty mountains filled my heart with longing. I dismissed it as an unconscious need for escape from our difficult circumstances and a long, cold winter. As it persisted, I took it more seriously and shared it with Bruce. He too, had sensed God tugging to a country with warmer climates, yet he enjoyed Canadian winters.

Once again we opened our missions file and re-applied for training as long-term crew with Mercy Ships. Like a prisoner losing hope of long-awaited parole, our expectations were set low.

This time Mercy Ships accepted our applications immediately. However, we felt reluctant to begin raising support from churches, family and friends. Already dangling on the edge of a financial cliff, we hesitated to plunge and trust God for our finances. Wrestling with a 'beggar mentality', we worked through a study guide, which confirmed the scriptural view of missionaries and pastors relying on the body of Christ for their needs. It seemed a tough thing to attempt in a culture where financial independence is closely linked with esteem. I felt uncomfortable putting people in an awkward position of obligation by asking them for a commitment. What if people lacked this biblical view? How would they view us? Scripture was clear and I would have to learn to release my fears into God's hands.

We followed prayer and fasting with a letter to family and friends stating our needs. Within six weeks, pledges for the $17,000 needed for our five-month training period came in! Buoyed by this confirmation of success and answer to our prayers, we firmed our plans to sell our home and many of our earthly possessions. The resurrection into our spiritual destiny finally seemed to be within our grasp.

Almost. One final death lay just around the corner.

Pines and Myrtle

Our heaped up mini-van resembled the Beverly Hillbillies as we prepared to set out for the US border. In April of '97 on a warm spring evening, church friends gathered to say farewell and pray for our family's journey.

Our children, now ages 9, 8 and 6, had resisted the possibility of missions two years earlier. Leaving grandparents, friends, our cat Jasmine, bikes, and their secure home was a sacrifice beyond their ability to make. We agreed that God would have to change their young hearts through prayer. The change appeared remarkable. Their excitement on this journey could hardly be contained! Mission bound, our destiny awaited at the Mercy Ships Crossroads Discipleship Training School (CDTS), Texas, USA.

Barriers became familiar to us in the journey of our dreams. We met our first at the Canada-US border. Customs officers weren't prepared to let this keen homeless family enter the USA. With gruff voices, the barrage of questions began. My heart pounded with fear as Bruce explained our purpose to disbelieving ears. Visions of returning in humiliation after just two hours from leaving home threatened harshly. Evidently we needed proof of financial support during our educational training.

Praying madly as I bounded to the van, I dug for our file box. With shaking fingers I produced proof of financial support from our list of partners and donors. Following 25 gruelling minutes of uncertainty, in sudden swiftness the officers' countenances changed and they granted entry. Turning to our children, with great conviction the officer added, "You kids are pretty lucky going on such an adventure with your parents—seeing the world." Reflecting on the officer's comments, Brandon thanked us as we crossed over the US border. They've never forgotten that viewpoint.

Three days later, as the hills bloomed and shouted of springtime in east Texas, our excitement grew by the minute as our journey drew us nearer. The gates of Mercy Ships International Center embodied our dream. Beyond them, lay our new home for the next three months. Met by the warm southern hospitality of our leaders, we relaxed and settled in.

Shortly thereafter, I became aware of the tall, beautiful pine trees surrounding the family dorm. Soft needles lay everywhere. I recalled the directional verse about pines and myrtle growing. Curiously I sought out the gardener at the green house on the base. When I asked him whether myrtle grows in Texas, he claimed they grew both in parts of Florida and Texas. "In fact there are several trees in front of the dining room and many lining the boulevard entrance to Mercy Ships," he announced!

Confirmation of God's leading! The dream had begun. I was certain.

11
Death at the Crossroads

> *These have come so that your faith—of greater worth than gold, which perishes even though refined by fire—may be proved genuine and may result in praise, glory and honour when Jesus Christ is revealed.*
>
> *I Peter 1:7*

It happened near the end of our three-month lecture phase. One evening, Bruce came hobbling to the dorm after playing volleyball. Familiar with this old knee injury, he knew that within several hours or days, it would click back into place. But this time he experienced no relief. Examinations revealed the need for surgery from a torn cartilage. He hobbled on crutches from building to building on the sprawling base.

For some time we prayed asking God where and how to have surgery at this inopportune time in our lives. We had often joked with fellow Christians about God sending a postcard from heaven to give divine guidance. On the day we prayed for guidance regarding location for surgery, an actual postcard arrived in the mail that astonished us. An older praying woman from our church sent a short note on the back of a postcard from Seaforth, our hometown. Several historical sites in Seaforth, Ontario would make lovely postcard material, but this one was an uninteresting photo of the Seaforth Hospital!

We eventually regarded it as the answer to where Bruce should pursue surgery. Rates for operations in the USA made it out of the question for us, so this made sense. With a free airline ticket from the air miles of a generous fellow classmate, Bruce flew back to Canada alone. A 10-day separation felt like weeks. Anxious to re-unite, the children and I scanned through streams of unloading passengers at the airport. Finally he emerged in a wheelchair pushed by a flight attendant. His embrace felt warmer than ever, a raging fever burned in his body. I joked uneasily that he gave new meaning to the term "hot lips."

Back at the base, his health continued to seriously decline. The violent, continual retching caused serious dehydration and stomach valve damage. Unexpected test results shocked us: acute Hepatitis C, the new dreaded disease—one with a stigma similar to AIDS. Bruce's lifestyle had never lent exposure to this type of disease. Nevertheless, we avoided the futile road of pondering the source when what we really needed was answers for the future. When the doctor strongly advised against our mission trip to Trinidad, the gates to Mercy Ships closed shut. Our dream locked out!

We had left everything: our home, our pet, our family, and our friends. In a state of brokenness, everything had been sacrificed to follow God's leading. Desperately wanting to trust that there was

Chapter Eleven

purpose for it all, we believed that a destiny lay just ahead. Now, in the midst of spiritual healing and grasping His deep love for us, it had all blown horribly off course.

Seeking a quiet refuge to sort through my pain, I tucked the children into bed and headed to a dark, quiet classroom in the family dorm. Thoughts of the kid's disappointment rushed in, releasing deep mournful wails. I loved their excitement as they prepared for Trinidad with tambourines, banners, dramas, and dance. I couldn't fathom breaking the news to them that we would not be going. The wailing turned to wrenching sobs. I struggled for breath.

While my husband lay ill, I faced the darkest hour and greatest crisis of my faith. Alone. *Was this God's idea of some kind of cruel joke? Bring us to the edge of release and then withdraw the dream? Did He not call us into missions? Is this not what He had been preparing us for all along? Why did He never allow anything to work out for the Meyers' family? Is God even really there?*

In those moments, all that I'd been taught and believed since childhood, all the faith that I'd developed through the years seemed to hang in the balance. Faith—shaken to the core by years of accumulated struggle and one final crushing blow of deep disappointment with God. An unbelieving friend once said that I had created this "god-life" in my head, like a child with an imaginary friend or playmate. Maybe he was right. God may be real, but all my experiential evidence pointed to this verdict: although He may run the universe, He must not play an active, loving role in the lives of individuals. Once again, I could choose to follow this God at a safe distance in fear and distrust. In fact, why would I desire to be close to a God who kept hurting me over and over again? Like Job's wife suggested, I could choose to "curse

God" and let my spiritual life die.

I thought I'd finally figured out this Christian life. Hadn't I learned that the key to God's blessing and favour on our lives was obedience? The fulfilling of our mission dream had been proving that. Since that key now seemed to have no guarantees, I felt lost in a maze of confusion with no way out. Helpless, I gave up the search to understand. Wrapped tightly in a fetal position, I wept, letting the doubts sit heavily. Eventually numbness silenced the pain.

Then, gently, as though pouring soothing oil, the Holy Spirit warmed my sorrowful heart. I felt powerfully drawn by an irresistible force to this God of pain and suffering. Comforted, I lay limply on the floor in quiet surrender. I decided then to trust Him anyway. The small voice whispered ever so clearly. "Though He slay me, yet will I trust Him."

Clinging to my renewed learning about the character of God, I repeated over and over:

God is good and all His ways are just.

God is good and all His ways are just.

But our dream of sailing to the poor died in the darkness of the family dorm.

Stage Six - Potter's Highest Fires

Temperatures in the kiln are set at their highest in this final stage for the clay pot. The fire becomes a brilliant yellow to cleanse away any impurities. Dampers are closed and oxygen is cut off from the kiln. Heavy black smoke follows and soot consumes the vessel.

As the highest fires burn, the purging for the Christian begins. Pride, position and competition are being consumed. The intensity and pressure is so great that we cannot hear or see comfort of friends and intercessors. Naked and choking in the smoke of the kiln, we feel lost and confused. The high fires leave us stripped of self, pride and reputation. Then slowly the Lord opens up the dampers allowing fresh oxygen to fill the kiln.

For us, the hope of entering missions had breathed new life into our broken, weary spirits. Then to our shock, our dream was cruelly snuffed out at the threshold. Seared by the hottest flames, I gave up my right to understand and let the dream die.

At the time I didn't appreciate that in the black fire, beautiful colours are pushed deep into the clay. These are formed only in the darkest hours of agony, grief and death.

12

Triumph in Trinidad

Ask of me, and I will make the nations your inheritance, the ends of the earth your possession.   Psalm 2:8

While the dream died, the old lies returned and invited me to dance. *You're not worth loving, Marilyn. Somehow you're not quite good enough.* That twisted and tarnished part of my life filter re-surfaced. I took up the dance, but only briefly. In the atmosphere of faith and love at Mercy Ships, other partners of the new dance proved stronger. One teacher expressed an image of me in a white flowing dress dancing with joy before the Lord. The evil lies slinked away.

My heart longed for a miracle. One that would wake me up and tell me it was only a bad dream. I felt twinges of pain as classmates talked excitedly about the outreach, but I also felt buffered and anesthetised by the hands of the Master Potter. Hands that kept the clay pot from exploding in the fiery death of the kiln.

Despite the uncertainty, we continued to meet with our Trinidad team. Our class members divided into two teams, as they felt led by God. One team prepared for Nicaragua, while the other set its sights on Trinidad.

Over the next week, the Trinidad team earnestly sought the will of God on our behalf. We dared to hope. Just a few days prior to departure, the decision was reached and together we agreed. Despite US doctor's advice against it, we would continue on and fly to Trinidad along with the rest of the team. Bruce seemed well enough so we entrusted his health into God's hands. He could recover while assigned with the role of prayer intercessor —the watchman on the wall based on Ezekiel 33 and 22:30.

> I looked for a man among them who would build up the wall and stand before me in the gap on behalf of the land.

The team warmly extended their hands and arranged last minute travel plans. As our destiny slowly resurrected from the grey ashes of death, we welcomed it guardedly and gratefully. Hope had been restored to us.

The Apprentices
Nineteen apprentice missionaries wore turquoise team t-shirts for easy identification in the crowded airports. Wearily we trudged off the plane in Port au Spain, Trinidad after a full day of travel and transfers. Bruce tired easily on the journey but the team patiently endured his frequent rest stops. Our youngest team member, Jessica, was a 16-month-old toddler whose parents also needed rests.

Abruptly a heavy wall of tropical humidity struck our senses as we disembarked from the plane. Noise and confusion reigned. Black faces stared. Shouting porters grabbed our bags against our

Chapter Twelve

will. Taxis roared off into the rainy night. Brandon became overwhelmed to the point of tears. While Bruce gathered our luggage, I tried to keep the kids together and calm. Fear filled their eyes as they tried to take in this new order of life, or lack of it.

Partnering with a Trinidad church from the town of Endeavour, transportation in Volkswagen vans had been pre-arranged along with our living quarters. With that, the nightmare trip of our lifetime launched a series of cultural surprises. Crammed into the Volkswagen van, we discovered no seatbelts and very few seats. The children were forced to crouch on the floor. Each time a car's headlights aimed toward us from the right hand side of the road, we gasped and braced ourselves for a crash. We froze with fear as the man in the left front seat hung his head out the window or turned around to talk to us. It made sense that he didn't watch the road when we finally realized the driver is seated on the right side of the van for left-side-of-the-road driving. Still, Frank, our driver, turned out to be more of a maniac racer.

With narrow misses and screeching stops, the unbolted seats slid forward and nearly crushed the kids on the floor. Bruce made the error of finding a seat near the back. A combination of heat and small spaces was a phobia that he had never quite conquered. Gasping with anxiety, he quickly opened a window and hung his head out in the rain for air and space.

Chadwick, who struggles with carsickness on hilly, winding roads, began to feel ill. We sent a message forward to the driver and he pulled over. On that dark, rainy night I stepped outside onto foreign soil to accompany Chad as he settled his stomach.

When we miraculously arrived in one piece at our Trinidad home, a host of smiling black and brown faces shyly greeted us. Graciously we accepted their handshakes and warm hospitality.

Approaching 11:00 at night, we all suffered from travel weariness and needed to crash into bed, but we lingered to fellowship with our hosts. Our children held up amazingly well, strengthened by prayer.

To make matters even more interesting, the women of the church had prepared a complete meal for us and motioned us to sit down at the table. We had no appetite, having already enjoyed supper on the plane and now we faced a dish of food set before us that resembled nothing familiar. Again, we consented and cautiously tested the food with smiles of gratefulness.

Bruce feared stories about eating rat and felt grateful it turned out to be chicken. We discovered that chicken prepared in a curried sauce was the main staple in the Trinidadian diet. To us it appeared as though the chicken parts had been separated with a stick of dynamite. Very little meat clung to those tiny bones.

Our new Christian 'Trinnie' friends sacrificed three of their own beds for the missionaries. Offering them to the eldest members of our team, we then appointed rooms accordingly on the upper floor of the island home. Wall-to-wall mattress and foam filled our cement-walled room. Settling in the next day, we found creative ways to hang wet towels on a makeshift clothesline above our beds. Following the example of other team members, we designed shelves out of wood and cement blocks to organize our living space.

Brandon, our oldest child, keenly felt the stress of being in a new country. As he awoke that first morning to the sounds of tropical birds, the beauty of lush green palm and banana trees, his distress faded into joyful anticipation. Sunshine on the world created a whole different perspective, but he never forgot those first terrifying hours in the darkness of Trinidad.

Chapter Twelve

Nine missionary children explored our new surroundings from within the grey, cement-walled compound. Naturally, the boys freely welcomed the new house pets of ants, flying frogs, bats, lizards, huge cockroaches and fist-sized spiders. Jillian, who recently turned six, quickly voiced her opinion on these matters. "This is a creepy country," she announced with disdain. Inwardly I echoed her sentiments.

Trusting her parents, Jillian walked the dusty, rutted roads through this "creepy country" into the town of Endeavour. A welcome service prepared by the church was being held in our honour.

Mangy dogs, squawking roosters, rank sewage ditches, staggering filth, and unthinkable poverty greeted us along the way. And this was only a partially developed country, or previously known as second world. Could it really be any worse than this in other parts of the world? This route became familiar as we walked into town daily, but we never grew accustomed to sights of poverty along the way. Reaching a part of the path that became difficult to pass after a heavy rainfall, the children termed it lava land because of the crater-like mud.

One evening, having left the church service early to put the kids to bed, the full moon shone high above the palm trees. As it shadowed over lava land, it lent the illusion of being on the moon's surface. How foreign this culture seemed to me—as faraway from home as being on the moon. As I raised my face to its beaming light, I remembered that our loved ones gazed at the same moon thousands of miles away. And it was comforting to know, that in this country of a thousand gods, we were connected to our family and friends by worship and prayer to the same One True God; the One who created the moon and this vast earth and sky.

Our Trinidad Inheritance

Spending hours with the local pastor, our team leaders discerned the areas of greatest need. As is the practice, Mercy Ships had not given us an agenda before entering this country. Part of our training was to learn to seek God and discover His leading for ministry. Walking in faith, not leaning on our own understanding and our own agendas can be a stretch for many Christians. Others perceive it as an exciting adventure!

Our vision became two-fold: to strengthen the local church of Endeavour and to reach out to the people of Trinidad with the love of Christ. A primarily Hindu people of East Indian descent and a minority of African people made up the population.

Our own Mercy Ships children polished their ministries on the balcony of our team's home. They used tambourines, ribbons, worship flags and dramas. Back in Texas, we'd been taught about the unique power of missionary children. We came to understand this in Trinidad. Local people seemed baffled by the fact that children of a rich culture travelled with their parents to live among them. One day a woman approached Jillian and me resting in the market area. She rubbed her hands slowly up and down Jillian's arm, intrigued by her fair skin. To many people it aroused sheer curiosity. Children opened otherwise closed doors and were considered a valuable part of the ministry. I appreciated the fact that Mercy Ships included and trained them rather than seeing them as mere tag-alongs. Like salt and pepper, our own children's white pale faces mingled amongst the dark faces of Trinidad kids.

Bruce, our designated watchman on the wall, still appeared gaunt, weak and thin. Nevertheless, he gained strength as each day passed. Feeling envious, he watched while the other men sweated it out in the construction of the church. Despite his physical weakness, he shone in areas of outreach to the community. A summer school organized in the mornings allowed him to use his teaching gifts. Children struggling to afford fees for regular school came to learn the basics of math and English each morning. On a wooden board painted black, he scratched out numbers and factors with chalk. Dried coconut shell hair served as his chalk brush.

Scheduled walks about the neighbourhood lent fine opportunities to visit and share with people in their homes. Evidently it became big town news that a team of white folk had come to them. They showered us with bananas and pineapples as gestures of kindness and hospitality. This reception of favour surprised us and reinforced the concept of missions for me. Foreign Christians can open doors that local ones cannot, simply because they are an anomaly in that land.

One day our paths crossed with Hannafa walking on the side of the road. She greeted me with a warm, lovely smile. Her delicate, sweet spirit captivated me. Hannafa, married to a man in his thirties, who years earlier beat her into submission, had eight children. She led me to her home—a dilapidated goat shack behind the middle class house of her brother-in-law. Apparently years ago a fight ensued between the brothers who shared the family home, resulting in Siri and Hannafa relegated to the goat shack. While the other wife remained childless in her spacious home, Hannafa produced eight "kids" in the goat shack. In the family home, the sister in-law devoted one room entirely to the gods. In it, a large shrine with Hindu paraphernalia served as an altar to worship their gods, while out back a family of ten survived in the cramped poverty of a goat shack. The injustice of it all angered me.

As the weeks progressed Bruce and I built a friendship with

Siri and Hannafa and their family. We learned that Siri had no permanent job to support his family. Bruce explored his desire for work, "If you had a dream what would you do for a job?"

"I would plant gardens and sell the fruit at the market." Siri gestured to his spacious grounds. Although an experienced gardener, he had no money for capital, namely tools, to begin his own business. Journeying to the market, together Bruce and Siri researched the possibilities for the best yield and return for crops. Using the team's outreach funds, Bruce bought the hoe, spade, gardening tools and seeds needed to get him started. By investing in this man's source of income, we could provide a long-term solution for his family's future. Our team left Trinidad before we saw the harvest of his labour. Bruce, the afflicted one, had not been expected to accomplish much in Trinidad. He felt blessed to have made a huge difference in a family's life.

As my friendship grew with the lovely, elegant Hannafa, I challenged her with the message of the gospel. On the balcony of our temporary home, overlooking grassy fields and mountainous rain forests in the distance, Hannafa prayed to receive Christ. I will always remember her beautiful smile and gracious spirit. Someday in heaven, I hope to meet again with the young woman who gave birth eight times on the dirt floor of her goat shack. Before we left Trinidad, we attempted to link her with women of the church.

Our church friends proved to be generous hosts. Desiring to give us a tourist view of their lovely island, they scuttled us off to Maracas Beach on our day off. We frolicked for hours in the salty ocean waves. Suddenly a mist rolled in over the lush, green mountains behind us.

And then I remembered. The recurrent mental picture of

green mountains and tropical mist that had persisted during our winter of despair was being fulfilled before my eyes. God had given me that picture, but I was too inexperienced to recognize his revelation to me. How awesome to understand this now. I revelled in the moment until the warm rains followed the mountain mist.

Palm trees silhouetted by the setting sun presented a tropical paradise that one might see on a travel brochure. We felt awed by the experiences that God granted us. Our eyes were being opened to the world. A beautiful, but lost world—one in which we might receive a small eternal inheritance.

Trials of Trinidad

With sweat dripping off his nose, Chris, our team optimist checked his fancy temperature-reading watch and declared that it was *only* 113 degrees Fahrenheit. Tropical heat proved to be a challenge for all us northerners. We welcomed the cooling, torrential rainfalls that poured down so furiously. Alas, minutes later the earth steamed up hotter than before.

As time wore on, the difficult living arrangements sometimes wore thin for our valiant team. Unity became challenged over trite issues, like a box of macaroni and cheese, and grocery lists. More serious issues arose like child discipline, safety, and how to spend our allotted budget. In a country of rampant wife and child abuse, and the confusion of a thousand gods of Hinduism, we marvelled that unity in the spiritual realm could be attained at all. We knew the spiritual battle against a team of evangelists would be great. Prayer, time in the Word and worship tools needed to be kept sharp and ready.

Sharing openly with our supportive team disarmed the distress from our struggles. Near the end of the outreach, I described my feelings regarding our time in Trinidad, "It felt like being confined in a filthy tin can, not wanting to touch the sides until I was safely airlifted out." Ashamedly, it revealed my position as survival, rather than adaptation to a new culture. But no one judged me. I believe they understood. I had a long way to go before becoming a true missionary. But it was a start for this refined, town girl from Baden, Ontario.

In boldness and trust we'd reached out to the saints of the church, the goat-shack family, drivers of flea-infested taxis, and the children of Trinidad. We offered friendship, encouragement, teaching and the love of God. Impacted, they had changed and we had changed. Nearly 200 people came to our home for a farewell celebration the night before our departure. Long, tearful farewells at the airport will always be remembered.

Boarding the plane back to Texas, Bruce's spirits ran high. He'd been granted a successful ministry in Trinidad despite his illness. His body gained strength over those two challenging months. Although he remained lean and easily fatigued, our watchman on the wall recovered significantly and triumphed in Trinidad!

13
Call Aboard

Like cold water to a weary soul is good news from a distant land.   Proverbs 25:25

With the Trinidad training behind us, once again I felt the anxiety of living on the edge, wondering whether God would leave us hanging. Disappointment, pain and uncertainty had become God's training ground for faith in my life. Stepping out in faith carried a deep price for one who likes to know what's ahead. Although I desired to trust Him for everything, part of me held back in fear. Admittedly, I still felt too vulnerable in God's hands after all the fires. *Would I ever learn to completely trust Him? Was I really strong enough to serve God as a missionary in a foreign land?* Despite my feelings, I chose to keep myself in a position of abandonment. In my daily quiet times, God's enduring love continually drew me to trust Him.

Arriving back in Texas, Bruce and I began to set our sights on a permanent mission location. The *Anastasis*, the largest of the

Mercy Ships fleet, had always been our dream. More recently, we had come to understand how unreachable that dream really was. According to one family, due to limited cabin space it could take years of waiting to get onboard! Instead Mercy Ships offered us temporary administrative positions at the Texas base while we waited for space on the ship to open up.

Spreading our net wider, we began contacting Caribbean YWAM bases in need of teachers, but with no tangible results. We agreed to begin work at the base that fall after a short return to family and friends in Ontario. Bruce had a slight sense that we would be going to the ship for a long time, so he felt a need to connect again briefly.

Homeless and feeling adrift, we returned to Canada that September. The beautiful maple leaf Canadian flag flying proudly at the border aroused the most patriotic feelings I'd ever known. Exuberantly, the children sang "O Canada" after our van passed through customs. We'd only visited one underdeveloped nation, but they had already learned to appreciate their home country.

A generous couple from our church offered us their home in Seaforth while they remained at their summer residence. Soon after settling in, we received the phone call from Mercy Ships which changed our lives. "Are you sitting down?" our friend Deb Potter asked, her familiar voice eager with anticipation. "The *Anastasis* desperately needs a high school English teacher and would like you to come to the ship as soon as you can!"

No other call would elicit such a joyful response from our family!
We cried!
We danced!
We embraced!

God was finally giving us our dreams after many long years of soul preparation. Through the dry winds and purifying, scorching fires of refinement we were learning to trust the One who had called us to Himself and loved us unendingly. God would sustain us as we lived out the dream.

Over the next few weeks, I stretched out my arms in trust even as small uncertainties arose in our departure process. We'd expected red flags about Bruce's health from the crew doctor aboard the *Anastasis*. Nothing appeared. Rather, *my* health condition became the cause for concern. We needed to send blood test results along with a doctor's note stating that my thyroid was normal and I could function under the stresses of ship living. Complying, we then waited patiently for the final acceptance and arrangements to be made.

Already learning to be flexible with our travelling missionary lifestyle, the children eagerly repacked their suitcases and bade farewell to school mates. We spent the final days with our family, knowing it could be years before ever seeing them again. Our contract with Mercy Ships only required a two-year commitment, but we'd left ourselves wide open to serving in missions for a lifetime should God lead us.

Finally, on October 5, 1997 at 2:00 a.m. eastern time, the Meyers family flew from Toronto to Holland, where the Mercy Ship lay docked for refit. Fully ablaze in our spirits, the dream kindled 12 years earlier was finally becoming reality. The uncertain transition time from the Potter's fires to the sea ended and a thrilling adventure lay before us. All aboard!

Stage Seven -
Potter's Purified Vessel

The purified clay vessel removed from the kiln is ready for its intended purpose. The shiny smooth surface emblazoned through the fires reflects the image of Christ. It is useful and prepared to carry wheat, fragrances, healing oils and living water.

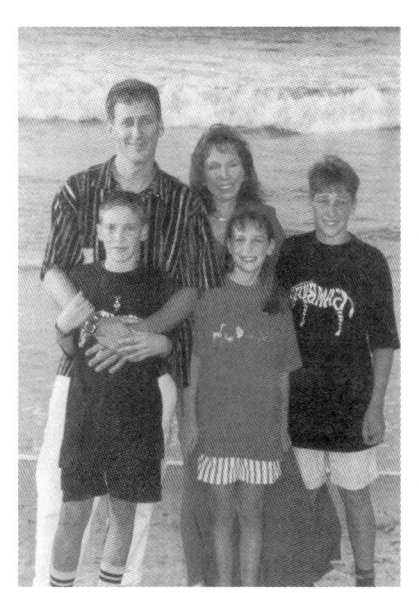

Meyers Family
on shores of Benin - 2000

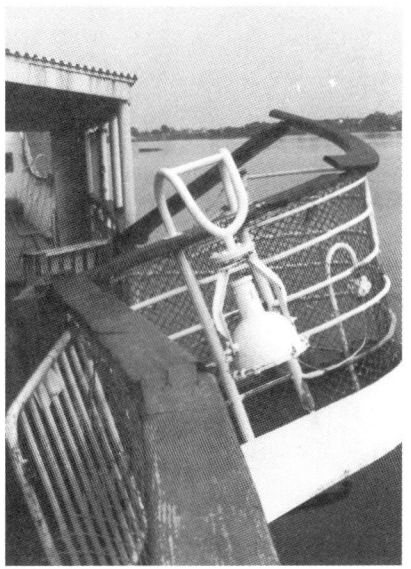

Damage to wing during
"touching" accident

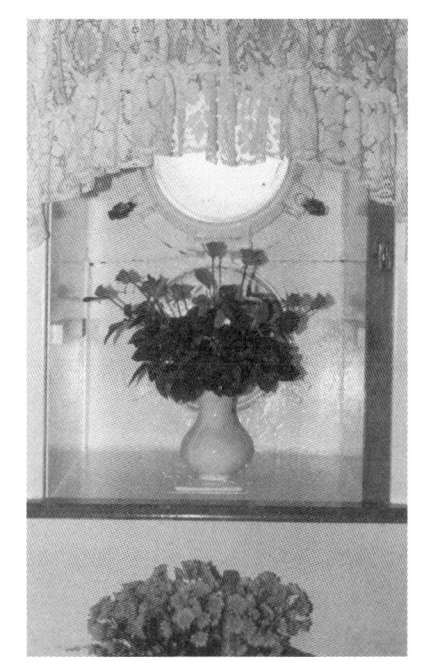

Painted porthole on C-deck

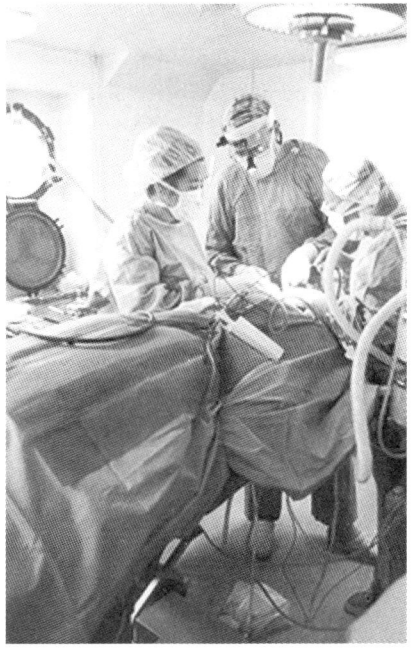

Surgery onboard

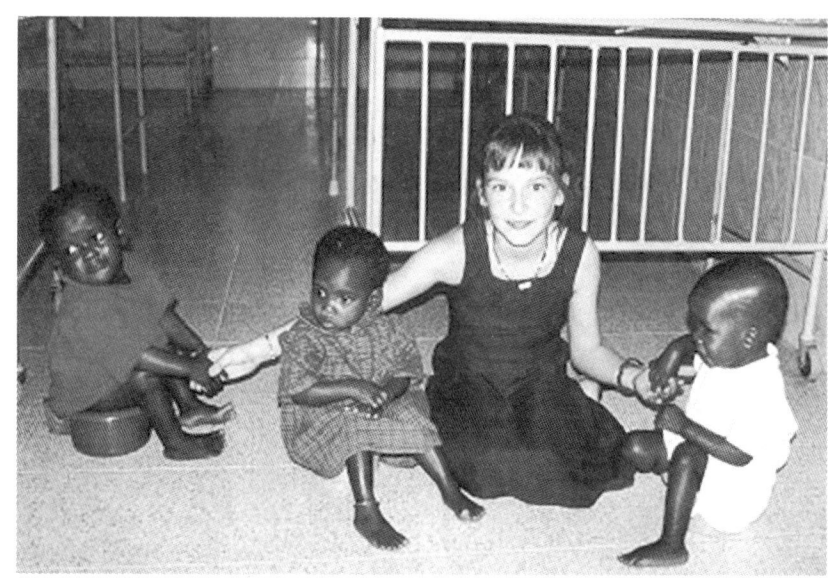

Jillian at the Sisters of Charity Orphanage

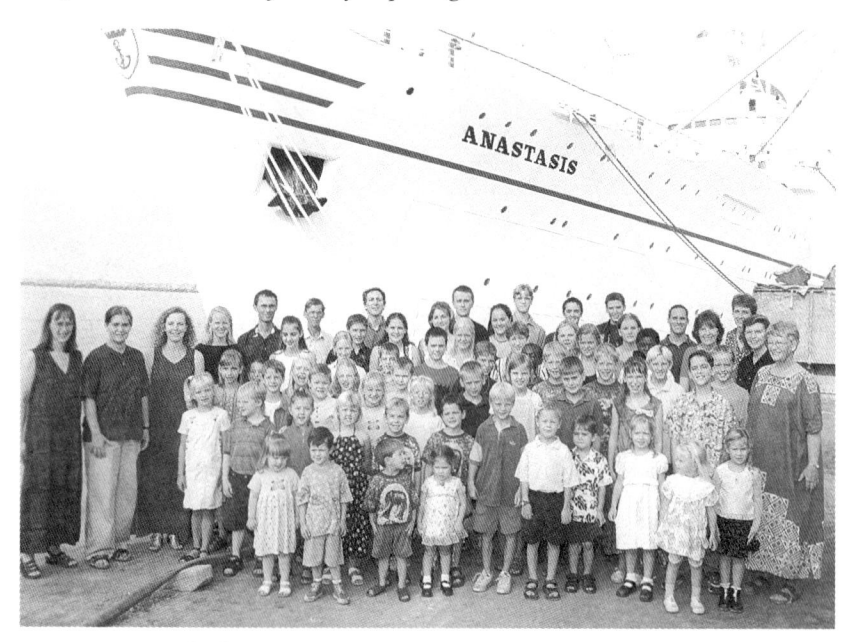

International Christian School in Benin - 2001

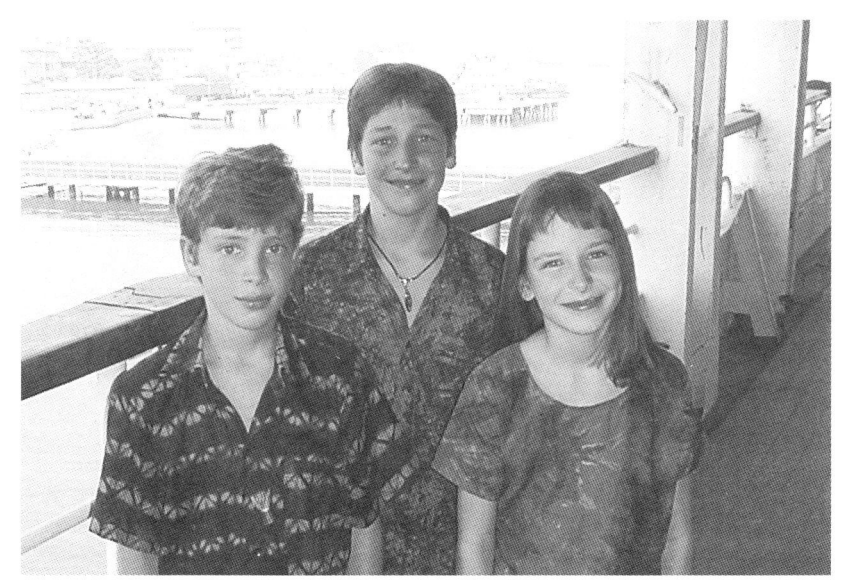

Brandon, Chadwick and Jillian on Promenade Deck

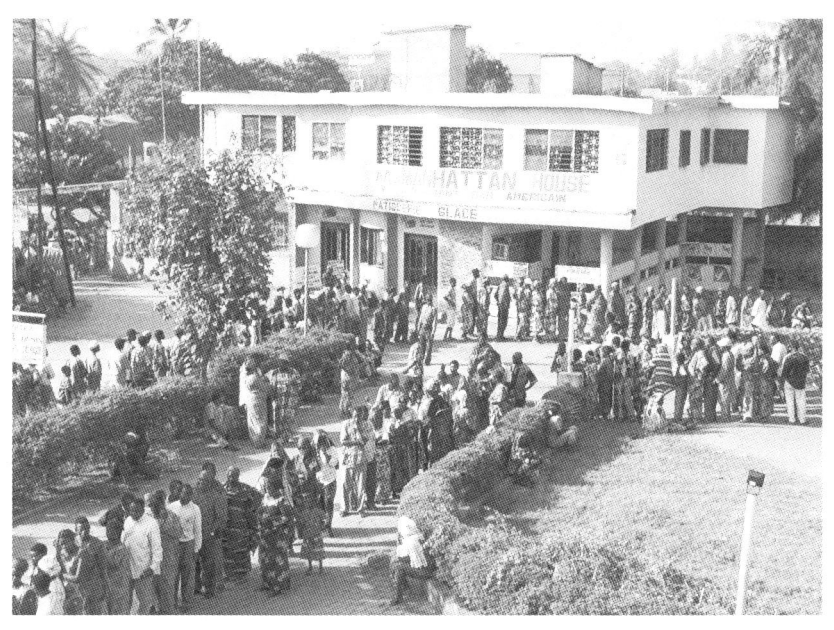

Screening day in Benin

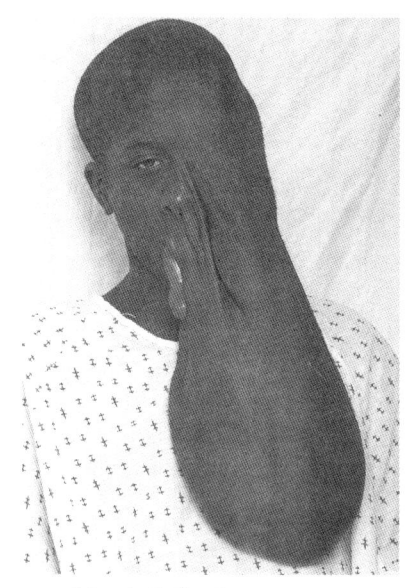

Mutala Before Surgery

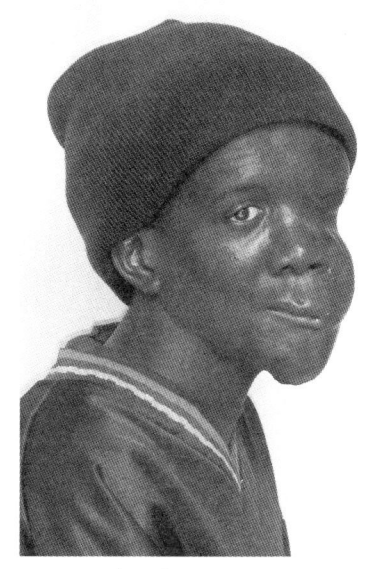

Mutala After

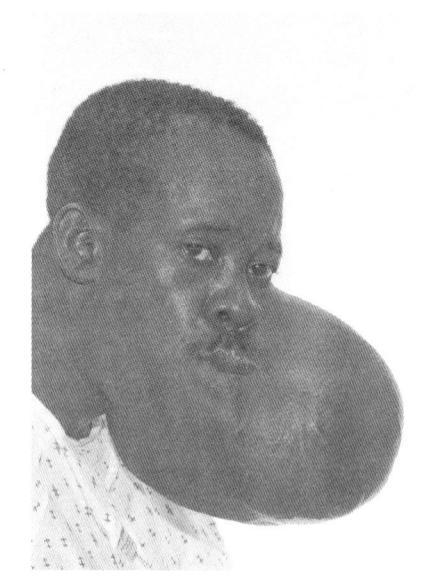

Malik Before Surgery

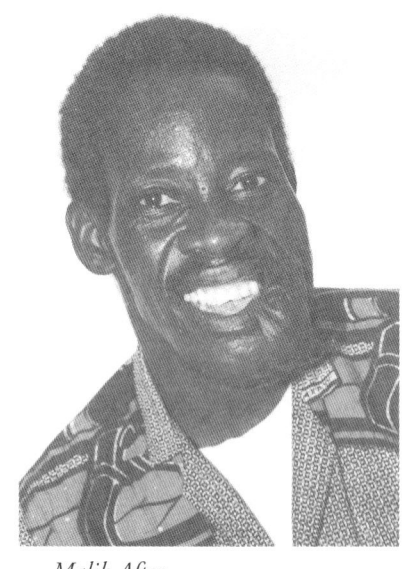

Malik After

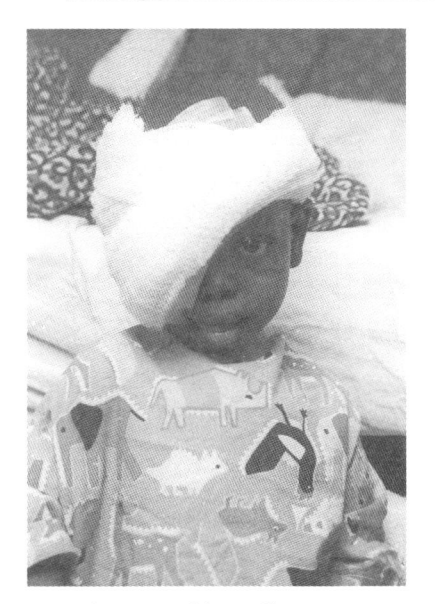

Three year old Cavilla

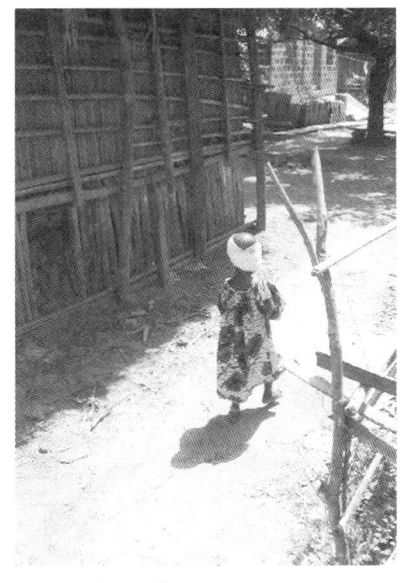

Cavilla's village

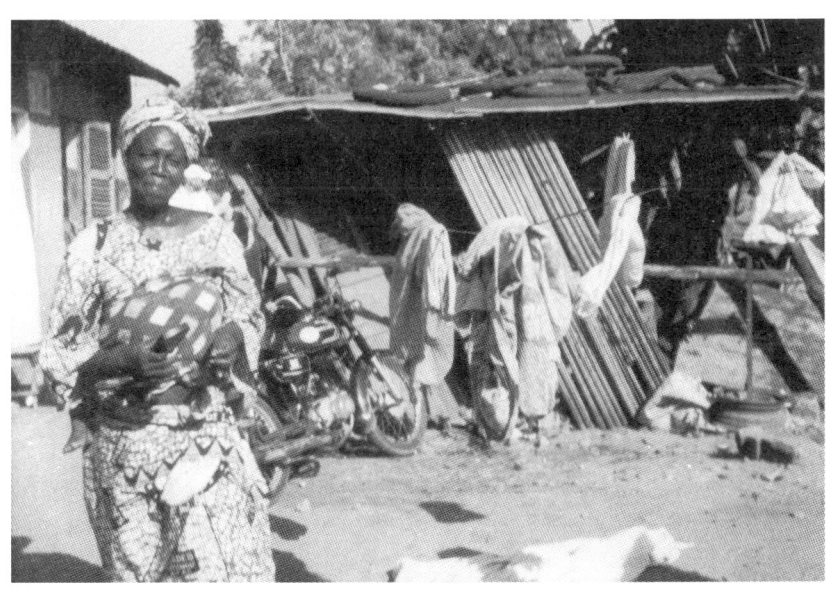

Widow Josephine in front of her hovel

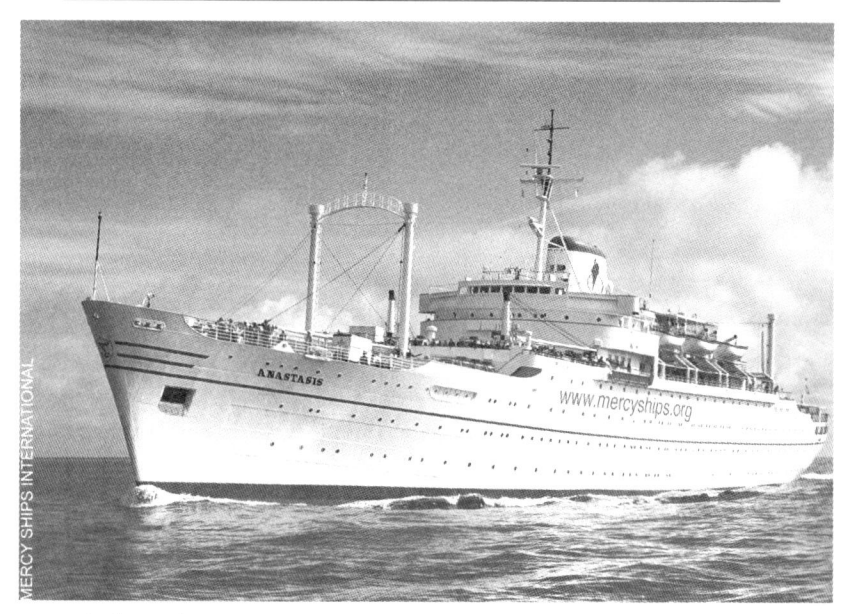

m/v Anastasis

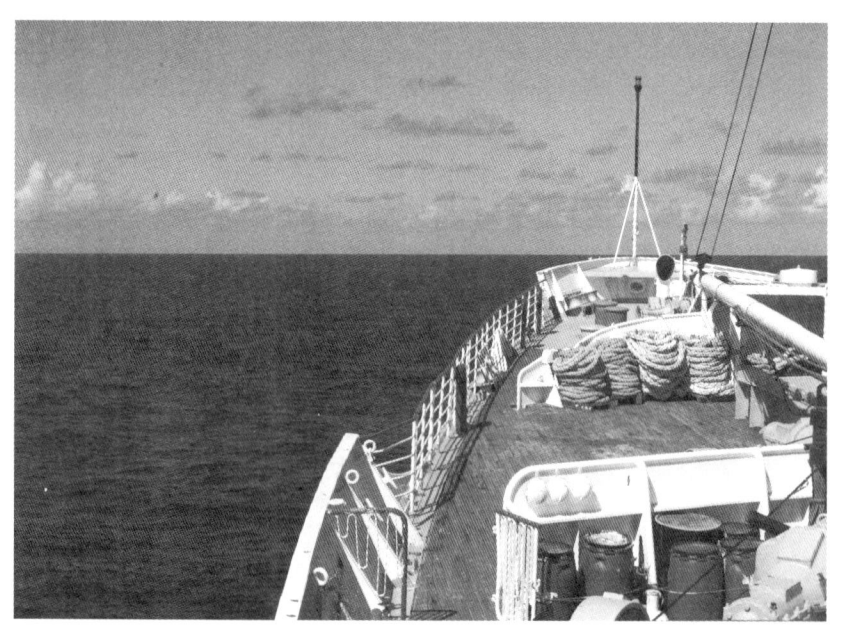

"Sailing is serene, marvellous beyond words."

PART II
Through the Sea

> *Your path led through the sea, your way through the mighty waters.*
>
> *Psalms 77:19*

14

painted porthole

> *Kings will see you and rise up, princes will see and bow down, because of the LORD, who is faithful, the Holy One of Israel, who has chosen you.*
> *Isaiah 49:7*

Partially pulling the shade on the golden October sun, I peered curiously below as the plane descended over the vast continent of Europe. Our future seemed to lie before us like the lands and oceans sprawling beneath. Unfamiliar and unknown. Distant and fascinating.

At the Amsterdam airport, we loaded our luggage into a rugged Land Rover owned by Mercy Ships. I imagined our family soon travelling on rutted, dusty African roads. While our vehicle darted past the dikes and windmills, our eagerness to board the Mercy Ship grew despite our tired bodies.

Slowly she came into view as we passed the gates to the port in Pernis. Looming high above the cranes and port structures, the tall crow's nest of the *Anastasis* guided us to our new home.

No longer just an image on a brochure or a dream beyond our

Chapter Fourteen

reach, she floated right before us—the world's largest non-governmental hospital ship. A massive vessel of steel and wood, she represented the symbol of hope and healing for tens of thousands. For us she symbolized the beginning of a long-awaited dream.

A slight scent of fish blended with the fresh channel breezes as we approached the narrow, temporary dry dock gangway. I hesitated slightly, assessing the safety of this unusual means of passage. Cautiously we climbed aboard as it swayed under our weight. I looked down briefly and gasped at the final steps high above the water. Only a few small steps left in this giant leap of faith, and at last, we crossed the threshold into Mercy Ships!

Safely inside, the lobby area surprised me. It seemed as though we had walked into a hotel foyer, with no sense of having embarked onto a floating structure. Impatient to see our cabin, I could barely focus my thoughts to complete the necessary embarkation forms. A friendly, uniformed receptionist talked routinely through instructions, fire drills and evacuation procedures. I tried to appear focused, but her words failed to lodge in my swirling brain.

Welcomed aboard by a Canadian host family, we followed them to our cabin, dragging our luggage one final time. For five and a half months we had lived from our suitcases. My nesting instinct had grown so strong that I figured any old corner could be made home for us. Or so I thought. Wending our way through the narrow passages of A-deck, down the stairs to C-deck, we headed for our cabin. In my heightened sense of awareness, I observed wires hanging from exposed deck heads (no longer would they be called ceilings) and men in hard hats with tools lying nearby. Dust and dirt made this old ship look more like a construction zone, which didn't fit the pristine image in my mind.

I had always thrived on order and cleanliness no matter how simple the surroundings. I'd always needed some element of beauty to survive. Not a great first impression. I would later come to know this as the dry dock or refit "look".

Finally we reached cabin 126 on C-deck port side. I had hoped for more, but prepared myself for less! The two-roomed cabin appeared shabby and small, but liveable, I decided at first scan. Immediately my eyes focused on a rusty porthole begging serious work. Then I sized up the tiny, unfinished makeshift table and decided it would make a better workbench for carpentry. With so little space in the room, there would be few meals together in this cabin.

A toilet and shower separated the two small rooms. Learning to step without tripping over flood barriers between rooms soon became a habit. The adjoining room for the children contained three ship-style bunk beds with green-striped privacy curtains. Having all three children in one tiny room would definitely be cozy living. Seemingly thrilled, they quickly staked out their beds.

Melanie, our smiling hostess from the hospitality department arrived with two jugs of orange juice and cookies. Never had I felt so grateful for fresh orange juice—something soothingly familiar and energizing.

A few weeks later, I fought tears as I returned to our wee cabin. I'd met crewmembers and viewed other family cabins. We definitely lived at the entry level. I remembered our lovely Seaforth home left behind six months ago. I pictured the soothing, antique green walls of the thickly carpeted living room, the stencilled ivy border in the hallway, the luxurious whirlpool tub in our ensuite bathroom. Our entire cabin would easily fit in the space of those two rooms.

I grieved the loss. I knew this day would come, and at that moment I became aware of the dangers of dwelling on comparison and looking back. Deep in my spirit, I felt grateful to be here, but could we really live out the dream in this place?

"Dear, you can make any place a beautiful home!" Bruce assured me. With those words, I set about the task. With help from Tina, the seamstress onboard, I re-covered the futon mattress that doubled as a couch and bed. Wide European-style olive green and white stripes instantly added character to the room. Accenting flowered pillows brought color and warmth. On good advice from another mother, I marched daily to the rear of B-Deck to the affectionately termed "Boutique." Filled with discarded items from crew members who ran out of space or needed to travel home lighter, the Boutique offered items free for the taking. For weeks, I dug for treasures to decorate our new nest.

During after-school hours, Bruce signed out tools from the carpentry shop to set about the tedious task of face-lifting the porthole and shower area. The war on rust began. While the needle gun pounded, our children happily explored all the narrow passageways of the ship, settling on aft deck, their new play area.

The end result satisfied us both. Lace Dutch curtains framed the newly painted porthole. Bruce delighted in the easily affordable prices of flowers in Holland and regularly bought me fresh bouquets for the porthole ledge. Cupboards began filling with basic dishes and cutlery. The countertop donned homey tin canisters matching the accessories in the room. The shower area brightened up with a fresh coat of white paint and a tiny rose-stencilled border. An inexpensive Monet print purchased in Rotterdam added the final touch to the barren walls.

It looked simple and small, but simple didn't have to mean

distasteful or devoid of beauty. My love for beauty and creativity had been a challenge in the past when coming to terms with materialism in our culture. Decorating our home and property without frivolous expense was the conviction I had followed for years. However, a tension to acquire more lavish living conditions existed strongly in North America. A media message of discontentment with our possessions and position in life silently corroded our biblical value system. Too often it found Christians bound unaware in the throes of materialism. Although I'd been content with our simple Canadian way of living, I would soon see how lavishly I had really lived when compared with our new home onboard, and then to the African friends we would soon meet.

Our nomadic family sighed in relief when Bruce finally stowed all our empty suitcases in the holds of the ship. Within a period of six months, we'd moved from Seaforth to Texas to Trinidad, and then briefly back to Seaforth. Having finally gone forth to the sea, at last we found ourselves living in a permanent home. Clothes which had been tightly packed in our suitcases hung neatly in closets or were folded smoothly into drawers. Stuffed toys found a home on shelves beside the kid's beds. With our cabin in order, we nestled in for the journey ahead.

A blackboard filled one entire wall in Bruce's little classroom. Scrounging through limited resources, he created colourful bulletin boards that stamped his personal fingerprint around the room. How Bruce had longed for this day—his own desk, his own teacher's daybook and his own students! Who would have known that his students would hail from various corners of the earth, representing many nations? Who could have imagined that his classroom would float around the world?

My position onboard remained a mystery for the first week.

Chapter Fourteen

When I received my assignment as secretary to the captain and deck officers, I felt honoured to serve alongside those in authority. Initially, my legs and heart protested the trek up to Lido deck starboard. I counted 70 steps from our cabin. At the top awaited a view worth climbing for! No land office window could match the view from my porthole. Deep blue sparkling sea and refreshing ocean spray often suspended my concentration on work and relaxed my anxious spirit.

Like Bruce in his classroom, I stamped my unique fingerprint in the deck office. To the amusement of the officers, I fastened a lovely straw hat with flowers and ribbons to the bulkhead (wall)—right beside the greasy hard hats of the "deckies" (deckhands). I quickly assessed the work cut out for me in this dusty, disorderly, office. Indeed it had been awhile since the deck department had a secretary to keep things in order. Experience had taught me to make changes slowly to a new work environment. However, greasy, strange looking parts, screws and fittings didn't belong in a paper tray and would require a new home quickly. I set about dusting shelves, books and manuals. Lastly I added a silk green plant to the porthole. Thankfully this porthole already appeared nicely painted. All this fussing probably mattered little to the men in this work environment, but it made a great deal of difference to me. They showed only slight amusement, until of course, the bosun (deck foreman) suddenly needed his mysteriously moved parts.

Princess Onboard

A taste of the public relations phase of Mercy Ships began two days after our arrival. Slowly the Mercy Ship moved out of refit and maneuvered up the channel to Rotterdam's prestigious downtown pier. From our porthole, we viewed the nightlights of the city reflected in shimmering colours on the water. Water traffic from tour boats and small craft created soft waves that lapped carelessly against the hull of the ship. The soothing sound would soon become as familiar as breathing.

Part of the awareness and fund-raising for Africa involved the scheduling of civic and press receptions, ladies' teas and youth nights. The professionalism of the volunteer crew in all these efforts impressed me. Day after day, smiling tour guides led long queues of people up the wide gangway and through the narrow passageways of the ship. Seeing strangers follow the tour ropes through our home felt both awkward and thrilling. I remembered that two years earlier we had toured the *Caribbean Mercy* in Toronto, another of the Mercy Ships fleet. The tour had affected me so powerfully that I fought to keep my composure. I longed then to be one of the crew members. As I reflected on this, my heart swelled with pleasure to realize that we now lived on the other side of the tour ropes.

A new buzz about the ship marked preparation for a momentous event—the arrival of Princess Margriet of Holland. To initiate the event, the founder and CEO of Mercy Ships, Don Stephens, encouraged us to be relaxed and allow the love of Christ to be evident in us. We'd made extra efforts to beautify the ship for this significant day. The media's presence would boost awareness and increase donations for the Mercy Ships service to the poor. All our nervousness for a woman of royal birth was understandable, but Don reminded us that we served the King of Kings and Lord of Lords. Some day every knee from every tribe and nation would bow before Him, confessing that He is Lord. In reverence and humility, our lives should reflect the King we serve.

Chapter Fourteen

Don's words put our jitters about meeting royalty into perspective. We prayed that the peace of Christ would pervade the ship and rule in us.

Captain Malcolm Carter from England saluted this honoured guest of royalty as she ascended the gangway. Excited ship children waved flowers from the rails of Promenade Deck. Dressed in a gold and black business suit, the lovely princess smiled serenely. Perplexed, Jillian questioned me, "Mommy, why isn't she wearing her crown and long dress?" This real-life princess didn't match her fairy-tale image of a princess.

The royal tour began with a rousing ceremony in the International Lounge, which seats 220 people. Due to her special interest in the school onboard, teachers and children waited expectantly in their classrooms, even though school had long since been dismissed for the day. Finally the princess and her entourage arrived in the Grade One classroom in the stern of the ship. The moment Jillian had been waiting for arrived! Shyly, she presented the princess with a bright bouquet of orange flowers on behalf of the ship's International Christian School. With a warm inviting smile, Princess Margriet bent down to talk with Jillian. Despite her youth, Jill felt the great honour of being in the presence of royalty.

Days following her visit, a letter from the office of the princess arrived. She expressed her genuine enjoyment of her visit and how the work and crew of Mercy Ships deeply moved her. Her aides commented that they had never seen the princess so relaxed as when she toured the ship. Perhaps the peace of Christ indeed touched her too.

It would not be the last time we would brush with royalty and presidents of nations. For our family, it had been an impressive initiation to the ministry of Mercy Ships in Europe.

A month after embarking we still found ourselves docked in the world's largest port in Rotterdam, Holland. Winds of winter blew stronger and colder. The Mercy Ship rocked in her berth as though impatient to depart. Down in C-deck, five new sailors grew eager for this unique missionary quest to begin, zealous to touch the lives of the poorest of the poor. With a sense of adventure, we prepared to navigate uncharted waters—our lives safely in the hands of our Heavenly Captain.

15
Forth to the Sea

The seas have lifted up, O LORD, the seas have lifted up their voice; the seas have lifted up their pounding waves.   Psalm 93:3

Everyone onboard warned us about the dreaded Bay of Biscay. They knew it to be the roughest, stormiest part of the journey southward from Europe to Africa. But only curiosity and excitement filled these new naïve sailors.

What does a large ship feel like in stormy weather? What is seasickness like? Were we true sailors or green-faced landlubbers? We soon discovered the answers to these questions.

Prior to this sail, work crews had installed upgraded fire alarms and sprinkler systems. This long phase of refit made everyone anxious to sail again. Communion and a unique "moving of the ark" ceremony ended this phase at the community worship meeting. I found myself deeply stirred at the depth of faith and abandonment to God's purposes shared by leaders and crew. This embodied the type of courage and faith that I'd longed to see expressed in the body of Christ!

Days before the sail, the atmosphere onboard transitioned as crew excitedly finished their work and prepared for the journey ahead. I set about learning how to secure the office computers, chairs and filing cabinets. In the captain's pre-sail orientation talk, he warned that we must no longer think in terms of horizontal surfaces remaining horizontal. "Objects placed on varying degrees of angles have a tendency to shift", Captain Malcolm stated with a humorously lecturing twinkle. He advised us to secure our cabins by fastening drawers, cupboard doors, and fridges with bungee cords or rope. Stereos and TV sets needed to be moved down to floor level during a sail. Hanging photos and picture frames could be sticky-tacked to the walls to keep them from swaying. The captain and officers then inspected work areas and decks for security before departure.

While mentally preparing for this unusual travel mode, I kept thinking I needed to pack suitcases or boxes. I couldn't seem to grasp this new concept that my entire home and office would be travelling along with me!

Everyone yearned for warmer climates on this unheated ship. Shivering crew in sweaters and parkas lined the Promenade Deck to bid farewell to Rotterdam friends. For seasoned sailors, they simply enjoyed another departure time, but for us, we faced our first time at sea! Our excitement could barely be contained!

Teachers suspended school schedules temporarily for the children during arrivals and departures. Piercing alarms jolted us all from our activities. "Attention all crew. Attention all crew.

Chapter Fifteen

This is the captain speaking. This is a fire drill. Please move quickly and carefully to your muster stations. I repeat. This is a drill. This is a drill," he articulated sharply with his charming British accent.

Routinely, departure from a port began with the pre-sail fire and lifeboat drills. During these practice drills, crewmen released winches and lowered lifeboats to Promenade Deck. Trained as a certified lifeboat crewman, Bruce worked bravely while his family silently watched. Although we practiced this procedure well over 50 times in the next four years, thankfully we never once had to board those lifeboats for an emergency.

Our family emergency bag tucked in a corner cupboard of our cabin should have made me feel more secure. Instead, I always found it disconcerting because of the constant reminder of the possibility of sinking at sea. I presume every sailor entertains images of going down, bobbing in life rafts for days, or worst of all, being swallowed by the ocean. These are images that a missionary sailor need not entertain when living in faith and abandonment to God's purposes, but admittedly, occasionally I did.

A last call for all staying ashore to exit the ship indicated that departure was imminent. With the gangway raised, phone lines cut, mooring ropes released, anchors lifted, the Mercy Ship floated smoothly and seemingly effortlessly away from the dock. Down in the engine room and on the bridge, a flurry of activity made it all possible. For the officers, sailing was often a long-awaited pleasure.

As required by law, a port pilot boarded to safely navigate us into deeper waters. The departure from Rotterdam in November 1997 is vividly remembered for the water gun salute from the two tug boats which manoeuvred us. Continuous fountains of water shot high into the air from the tug's water guns; a great honour for a ship to receive.

At first, we could barely tell she was moving. Only a slight rocking sensation could be felt as the banks receded. The deck rails emptied, as one by one, crew members resumed their normal ship activities. Hours from Rotterdam and well on our way, the pilot exited the ship by way of a rope ladder to his pilot boat.

This final procedure while underway provoked a strong sense of freedom and adventure in me. No more tours onboard. No more visitors. No more loading procedures. Only the Mercy Ship family, ocean bound and seemingly unreachable. Lost in a panorama of sky and sea. Eleven thousand tons of steel—only a speck on the vast ocean, held in the palm of our heavenly Captain's hands.

For several hours we experienced a taste of the gentle rolling that became a constant part of sailing. The passage to the English Channel increased the magnitude of the rolling sensation. Even for us new sailors, it was unmistakable when we'd reached the infamous Bay of Biscay.

Suddenly tempestuous, stomach-churning seas found the mid-ship Mediterranean Lounge littered with bodies trying to keep down their saltine crackers. With gale force winds near hurricane readings, the *Anastasis* became a battered ship in the midst of a storm. She rolled. She pitched. She corkscrewed. Massive waves pounded her bow.

Down in C-deck I perched on the porthole ledge to watch the stormy sea. At one moment the ocean held us high on a wave looking down to a rolling 30-foot trough of water. The next moment our porthole submerged into the ocean with water

Chapter Fifteen

swirling around it like a front-loading washing machine. It both fascinated and frightened me. I felt a sudden compulsion to keep my family close by.

Later that night a new razor-sharp fear gripped my heart and sent a wave of heat through my body. I envisioned one of our children sleepwalking (Brandon had a history of this in his early years) and quietly leaving the cabin. Walking dazedly to aft deck, he might climb the rails dreaming he jumped into a pool only to plunge into the dark, murky depths of the ocean. Lost forever. That horrifying thought recurred occasionally throughout our time onboard. I battled to release my children into God's hands. I reassured myself with the fact that Mercy Ships had taken great measures to ensure the safety of children onboard. Heavy orange mesh covered the deck rails to eliminate dangers for toddlers. In the 28-year history of the *Anastasis*, no one has ever fallen overboard.

Throughout the night, sounds of angry waves crashing alongside the steel hull kept me awake. In the darkness, I came face to face with the overwhelming fear of dying at sea. Not having land beneath my feet somehow made me feel totally out of control. What a false sense of security I carried in my life. *What made me feel I controlled my own protection and safety on land? If I truly believed God held my life in His hands, then what had I to fear if we should indeed perish that night?* Jesus said that not one sparrow would fall to the ground apart from the Father's will. Feeling absolutely vulnerable, I could only submit our family to the care of the ship's captain and to God's will. Peace calmed my heart as I handed over control to a trustworthy God.

It went on record as one of the fiercest, longest storms the *Anastasis* sailed through. Staying balanced proved to be a constant struggle and gave new meaning to the term drunken sailor. Only our first sail and how quickly I had grown weary of the battle against nausea and the fight against gravity. Had we only left the Potter's fires to face raging seas?

Halls appeared deserted since most people struggled to move about. By the fifth day of our first sail, work and school became sporadic. Bruce and Chadwick, feeling too unwell, couldn't remain in our forward cabin where the motion was greater. Instead they lay flat on the floors of the Mediterranean Lounge. Mirrored walls in this lounge still tinted slightly pink for the former cruise line passengers, tricked sailors into feeling well. A fresh pink look greeted us, as opposed to our true greenish colour.

Brandon and I discovered that we fared better when the ship pitched rather than rolled. Only two members of our family managed to stay well during the entire trip. Jillian and I boasted of having steel stomachs. On a later sail, I paid for my gloating when my husband teased me mercilessly after one episode of all-out seasickness.

While retiring for the night on Day Four of this rough voyage, suddenly the futon bed slid wildly across the floor. Simultaneously our cassette tapes, which I had packed tightly on the shelf, flew out and landed in a messy broken heap. Our damage appeared minor compared to those who had to replace their glass or dinnerware. To this day, crew members tell stories of the damage in their cabins and work spaces sustained from the one giant wave that sent us all to the starboard side.

My sleep grew fitful, broken by the sensations of floating one moment and being sucked deep into the mattress the next. Bumps, clanks and creaks in the ship shook the soundest of sleepers awake during a rough sail. Near our cabin, a steel flap allowing treated septic water to flow to the sea clunked continuously and rhythmically. Inside I screamed, "Stop this awful ride and let us off. Sailing is wretched, cruel beyond words!"

In the reception area, a tiny wooden ship on a large chart indicated the progress of our voyage. The further south we sailed, the smoother the seas became, until their lurching gradually ceased. Many began to feel human again and the once empty alleyways and decks slowly came to life.

Further south, the sea air steadily changed. Tropical humidity moistened our skin like a wet, sticky blanket. Winter coats appeared in the ship's Boutique. Sleeveless, cool cottons replaced woolly sweaters on deck. Faces glowed with perspiration.

Gloriously calm seas beckoned sleepy crew on deck to spot whales, dolphins and flying fish. When the bridge announced dolphins to starboard, teachers took their classes to aft deck to watch nature's show. Why study ocean life from a textbook when you can see it in real life!

From high on the bridge, an endless view of sky and blue sea soothed the weary sailor. Mirrored sunsets, a vast panoramic horizon bade worship of our awesome Creator. Sailing suspended our usual busy, western pace of work. The now relaxed, no longer seasick crew could admit—what a wonderful way to travel! I agreed, "Sailing is serene, marvellous beyond words."

From our secure small town of Seaforth, God had sent us forth to challenges and adventures on the sea. Although sometimes our experiences proved harrowing, mostly we sailed serenely undisturbed. We witnessed God's majesty and power roaring in the thunderous ocean waves and whispering softly in the gentle sea breezes. Flying fish, saucy sea gulls and delightful dolphins displayed the imagination and love of our Creator. With His painted sunsets, He seemed to bid us sailors goodnight. And with each new dawn we awoke to His mercies—new and fresh, shining like the rising, golden sun on the endless horizon.

Prior to this incredible voyage, a friend in Seaforth penned the following quotation in calligraphy.

> You cannot discover new oceans, unless you have the courage to lose sight of the shore.

How true that turned out to be. The safe shores of our town had been a splendid harbour in our lives, one not easily left behind. Our Captain God beckoned our family to distant new oceans, promising to keep us safe through fire and tempestuous seas. Without the assurance of His hand at the helm, we might never have left Seaforth and gone forth to the sea.

16

Fires, Riots and Pirates

> *The LORD will keep you from all harm—he will watch over your life; the LORD will watch over your coming and going both now and forevermore.*
>
> *Psalm 121:8*

Dangers of every kind could have easily overtaken us on this journey to the world's forgotten poor. Most times we remained naïvely unaware. However, as my experience in the deck office grew, I gained a stronger glimpse into what could happen. I had seen the official contingency plans ready for all times and occasions. Occasionally danger did strike closely reminding us of our unique lifestyle and vulnerability. The closer we came to harm's way, the more I wondered how many angels guarded us and protected the ship.

Guinea Outreach 1999

In Conakry, Guinea we discovered a country troubled by civil unrest. Tribal animosities and emotions ran high prior to the December national election. As the day approached, security measures tightened for our ship as well as the diplomatic community and ex-patriots. Evening curfews and shore leave changed.

A gathering of angry mobs was no place for anyone to find themselves, but even less, one with white skin. Demonstrating youth stormed the country with shooting, vandalism, riots and skirmishes. Like a hungry beast, these mobs mauled and killed recklessly, mercilessly with no regret.

One afternoon while returning to the *Anastasis* in a blue VW van, our family and a few crewmembers unwittingly encountered such a mob. Fear gripped us when angry, dark faces quickly surrounded us. Bodies pressed against the van as Bruce inched it forward and directed us to pray. Volatility threatened; we knew at any moment the mob could choose to rock and overthrow our van. Slowly and perhaps miraculously, we escaped through the mob unharmed.

During these critical times, the captain remained in touch with British and American embassies. Crew members confined to the ship checked the white board for reports. Day after day it read, *No shore leave*, followed by an update on riots and areas of alert in the city.

Although we cocooned safely aboard, we felt the heightened sense of imminent danger. The captain remained vigilant in his watch and commands to the crew. The safety of 400 people rested

Chapter Sixteen

in his hands. If the situation within such a country became too volatile with lives at risk, an emergency procedure to anchor at sea became the ready option. As a storm brewed on land, we felt secure knowing that our captain could navigate us to safer waters at any time. The grand ole' lady felt like a safe, roving refuge.

As riots eased up, the captain allowed shore leave with an evening curfew. Advised to leave in groups only and to avoid marketplaces completely, crew ventured ashore. Menacing tanks at major intersections reminded us that the city remained on edge.

On one occasion, the Mercy Ships Community Health Team returning to the ship narrowly escaped rioters who left police buildings and fire stations ablaze in their wake. Afterward, charred cement walls glared like festering wounds in parts of the city. The ship's teams returned home in awe of God's protection over them.

During these unstable times, it became vitally important to obey our captain's orders. Some crew members unacquainted with marine authority and accustomed to personal freedoms balked against the restrictions and foolishly placed their lives in jeopardy. They headed off to the market or restaurants as usual.

Seeing this, I understood why God sets limits in our lives for our own safety. When we disobey the Captain of our lives through a strong, independent will or recklessness, we take ourselves out from under His protective authority. In His mercy, often our Captain God will rescue us, but sometimes we bear the scars of this foolishness.

Rumours of pirate activity off the coast kept our officers and deck watchmen on guard day and night near the end of our time in Guinea. An Italian ship moored beyond the breakwater encountered the horrors of such an attack. Though within sight of our Mercy Ship, none of our crew saw the band of men with automatic weapons steal aboard. The captain, while held at knifepoint, was beaten for a ransom of $50,000. Pirates then ransacked and plundered the ship.

The Italian ship's crew managed to dock their ravaged vessel behind our Mercy Ship. They turned to our hospital ship for help. With great care, our medical staff freely attended to the wounded men—men greatly in need of mercy.

A week later, as we departed Conakry, we experienced a unique farewell. Standing on the deck of their ship, the Italian crew bound up in bandages and holding crutches in the air, saluted and waved. Their horns blared continuously. We returned the gesture, making it a noisy, memorable departure. A sailor's thank you—a sailor's farewell.

Republic of The Gambia Outreach 2000

Blaring fire alarms angrily roused us from deep sleep. "This can't be a drill!" I stammered after bolting straight up in bed. Routine drills never occurred at 2:30 in the morning.

"Quick, you get the boys awake and I'll carry Jill," Bruce instructed. Promptly I gathered the frightened boys while Bruce carried Jillian in his arms allowing her to continue sleeping. The commotion at the gangway and the night air woke her instantly. Bleary, but wide-eyed, we joined the other crewmembers clustering on the dock.

Alert in the ward, nurses and frail patients also prepared to evacuate. A serious hush swept over the anxious crew. Some huddled together to pray for God's intervention and for the firemen fighting the flames. Others seemed too stunned to think or pray, but stared in disbelief at the smoke billowing from the stack and the sparks spewing like fireworks into the humid night air of The Gambia.

Skillfully, courageously, fire teams doused a huge, spontaneous wood fire, birthed near the incinerator in the engine room. Only one hour and 15 minutes from the alarms, everything was under control. The nightmare ended.

Chief Engineer, Brandon Laing had been the first to awaken that unusual night. Thinking he heard alarms in the engine room below his cabin, he awoke to check his beeper. Baffled to discover his beeper turned off, he felt compelled to check things out anyway. Minutes later as he approached the engine room, the ship's alarms suddenly began screaming. A mysterious pre-warning had alerted him in his sleep, and prepared him to begin the necessary procedures to put out the fire. It had saved precious time in the battle against the flames.

That fretful night we embarked on the ship slowly, grateful for our lives and for our home. We had been saved by fire alarms, fire teams, the captain and a chief engineer who awoke in advance, ready to fight a fire. Once again, we had experienced God's miraculous protection through Chief Brandon's pre-warning of the fire.

Most certainly, it had been a night to remember. Nestling in again for the night, we hoped for sweeter dreams.

17
steel scars

I bear in my body scars from my service to Jesus.
   Galatians 6:17, The Message

The challenges of the sea were few, but highly memorable. I learned to overcome my fears for my children's safety onboard and of sailing through stormier waters. Having experienced storms at sea, a fire onboard and evidence of rioting and pirating, I was learning to deeply trust our Captain God for our safety. I had become accustomed to the unpredictability of a sailor's life with its ever-changing schedules and the element of adventure and surprise, but far from my consciousness was the remote possibility of an accident at sea.

En route to Benin for a seven-month field assignment, the *Anastasis* planned to deliver 20 tons of cargo to the Mercy Ships' New Steps team in Freetown, Sierra Leone. Meant to be a short stop with no shore leave, the deck department prepared to offload equipment, prosthetic limbs and supplies for this war-torn nation.

No tugs waited to safely escort us to our berth. In their bid to overtake the government, rebels had scuttled them. Built in the days before bow thrusters improved manoeuvrability, the Mercy Ship relied on the teamwork of the officers, engineers and tugs to safely dock. The pilot assured our Captain, a Master of multiple-class vessels, that no currents disturbed this harbour.

With only a few metres separating us from the dock, it

appeared that we'd arrived safely. Then from the rails of Promenade Deck, I witnessed one end of a mooring line snap forward and hit the dock with a loud crack, coil, and drop like a snake into the water. Had anyone been hurt? Suddenly the PA blared, "Emergency stretcher team to the bow!" This dreaded announcement meant one thing. The rope had hit someone! The crew chaplain, trained and experienced as a linesman, worked on the bow with the other men. When the line snapped, he became its victim.

Thrown off his feet, Perry Balcom sustained serious injuries to his leg. Flown to England, he underwent surgery on two fractures. Many considered it a miracle that he'd not been killed. Was it the mercy of angels guarding him that day?

The departure from Sierra Leone without the use of tugs proved to be even more dramatic than the earlier arrival. The scene unfolded on a sunny, equatorial day with the usual cheers from the dock and waves from crew lining the rails. A bulky rice carrier lay berthed behind us and a long breakwater of rocks in front. Pulling clear away from the dock, a good wide berth made our manoeuvre out to sea look smooth. Something changed. A current caused us to drift in, closing the wide berth we had gained. My husband turned to our friend from the radio department and announced matter-of-factly, "We're going to hit that ship."

It seemed too soon to tell, but as we continued to drift in, he reiterated that fact. By now crewmembers strained from the railing to look for clues from the captain on the wing. He remained calm with his radio in hand. Moments before impact, I remained in disbelief that we would actually hit. I had come to trust the captain implicitly and naïvely thought no harm could beset us on the Mercy Ship.

Chapter Seventeen

It's called a "touching" in marine language, a common occurrence. Unlike land accidents where there is impact, followed by an abrupt end, this seemed to go on forever. Our hull scraped along a considerable full length of the massive carrier. Only a touching—but the sound of steel scraping steel will remain forever locked in my memory.

Debris began to fall from Lido Deck and crew scurried back from the railings. Our mild-mannered CEO and chief surgeon, Dr. Gary Parker, yelled firmly for people to move back. Look-out wings heaved and bent their shape, railing contours twisted and steel floors bulged up. Lamps on the side of the ship were flattened like pancakes. A young African man aboard the carrier threw a flattened lamp back to our ship. It landed with a heavy thud on Promenade Deck. Then we watched his face as he witnessed the damage unfold. As the horrible screeching continued, he held up one finger, then two, indicating damage to two lifeboats. We grimaced as we looked into one another's faces. Aghast and speechless, we stood helplessly waiting for it all to end.

Suddenly the bosun leaped down from Lido deck commanding and herding the crew quickly to the aft deck. The screeching stopped and we began drifting out slightly, then back in once again. It appeared as though round two of this nightmare was about to begin. Anne, a Norwegian friend began praying for a wind to move us away.

To make matters worse, the captain received word from the engine room that the engines were running severely low on air, limiting potential manoeuvrability. At that precise moment, the captain's simple prayer for wisdom was answered. Captain Ketchum shares his perspective on that fateful day of November 3, 2000:

So - there we were. Rocks ahead, limited air, dock to starboard, a ship behind, a potent current, the pilot shouting, two lifeboats gone, platforms buckled, railings damaged. It was there and then that I felt the grace of God upon me. I had an immediate and very clear sense of exactly what to do to get us away. It was as if everything became hushed. I issued a few orders... and we came clear, into open water.

In looking back, I see so strongly God's hand of protection. At one point we were in a dangerous position, but we came out of it with damage which was fundamentally cosmetic, no harm done to the superstructure or the propellers.[1]

In times of danger, I discovered that it became urgent to have my family nearby. Brandon had courageously rescued the third officer's young son who became paralyzed with fear at the impending danger. People shouted for him to come away from the aft wings, but Brandon acted quickly by grabbing him seconds before we slammed. Jillian had been playing with friends on aft deck and came running to us. We were all accounted for, except for Chad.

My heart seized with fear. Why wasn't he with the other children on aft deck? Had he been close to the danger? Brandon began to check all his regular haunts about the ship and soon found him in the captain's cabin. Not a concern in the world, he happily played computer games with the captain's sons, Ben and Will. The boys had heard some strange sounds, got up and filed down the Lido deck passageway. They sighted the captain and viewed some damage of the deck and rails. Unconcerned, they returned to their games.

I didn't know whether to laugh or cry. Oh, the simple trust of children. *Could we ever respond like this in times of crisis?* If we would take a glimpse of our Captain God, see that it's all under control, and then carry on with life, we could save ourselves a host

Chapter Seventeen

of needless anxieties.

Naturally, out of my fear, I scolded Chad for this bad habit of forgetting to inform us of his whereabouts, especially during sails. He often became engrossed in play with his friends and lost all sense of time and responsibility. How many times I had fretted and marched the corridors looking for one of my children! I determined that stronger consequences needed enforcing as a safety measure for the whole family.

Passing the breakwater, we sailed away from the harbour into open coastal waters. Here we anchored safely to assess the damage. In shock, crew wandered the decks aimlessly. A member of the chaplaincy team stood on the mounted anchor of aft deck and prayed with difficulty. We ended with a chorus. People remained silent, tearful and prayerful. An obvious, but unspoken question loomed loudly. With all this damage, could we sail to our destination and its people: the poor of Benin?

Anchored offshore in dangerous waters for the night, we awaited word from our insurers, Lloyd's of London, regarding our damaged lifeboats. Hundreds of crew members might be flown from Sierra Leone to Benin should we not be given permission to sail. The final word came. It was deemed safer to sail than to fly crew out of an unstable country like Sierra Leone. The captain shares his account of the pivotal hours that followed:

> Had lifeboat 5 been taken out like the other two, our mission to Benin would have been in serious jeopardy. In order to sail on to Benin, we needed additional life raft capacity for 76 persons. And here we discovered yet another provision of God—taken onboard three years previously and stored in the hold—four fully operational life rafts with a capacity of 80. We were more than taken care of. We were sailing with a crew of 340 and have life saving capabilities for 541 people.

This was God providing in abundance and showing His hand of mercy toward us.

The following morning, after anchoring out, I went by the pilot boat to visit the Ekuelle captain and the Freetown Port authorities. There, once again, I saw evidence of the grace of God. The Ekuelle's captain received me with warmth, genuine concern, and kindness. He waved away the rail damage to his vessel as "minor", certainly nothing to be making claims about. Our ship being all white (and beautiful), he thought we were a tourist cruise liner. We talked about the mission of Mercy Ships, our history, our name. I could hardly believe it when he told me he was Greek. And his name—Plomaritis ANASTASIOS!

And finally, in the Harbour Master's office about seven other port officials had assembled. After expressing their commiseration, to my surprise one pilot asked if they could pray for us. Next thing I know, we were huddled—like in a football game. And pray they did—for the blessing of God upon our crew, our mission, our work. How amazing is our God! [2]

Another miracle! Once again, we perceived that God was showing us mercy as His Word declares. "Blessed are the merciful, for they will be shown mercy" (Matt.5:7).

A day later, while finally underway, we saw the lights of Sierra Leone piercing the dusky sky and shimmering on the ocean. Green coastal mountains render Sierra Leone one of the most beautiful West African countries. Our Mercy Ship had only been scheduled for a brief stop there, but our slight "touching" of this wounded, war torn nation had left its mark. Our ship bore deep steel scars.

We settled in for our final stretch of the journey. All was quiet, except for engines humming and ship walls creaking. The giant cradle rocked a weary crew to sleep.

Sometimes being a landlubber felt vastly safer.

18
Floating Village

> *May our dependably steady and warmly personal God develop maturity in you so that you get along with each other as well as Jesus gets along with us all. Then we'll be a choir—not our voices only, but our very lives singing in harmony in a stunning anthem to the God and Father of our Master Jesus!*
>
> Romans 15:5, 6, The Message

Like the international flavours of coffee, each new season brewed a unique, refreshing blend of nationalities aboard the Mercy Ship. Crewmembers from more than 35 nations blended as one. They flew to the Mercy Ship from Malaysia, Greece, Trinidad, Australia and New Zealand, Canada and the USA. They boarded her directly from the UK, Norway, Latvia, Holland, Germany, Ghana and Togo, Madagascar and South Africa.

Dividing walls between these nations were broken onboard the Mercy Ships. Over 400 people, from diverse cultures and walks of faith, live and work on floating masses of steel. With a mixture of skin colors, from the infant to the aged, they are all different, but blended and bonded by the spirit of Christ.

Like wafts of smoke from the ship's stack, the sounds of worship lingered over the deep Atlantic Ocean as we sailed together. I imagined them rising from the ocean as a sweet fragrant offering, then dancing lightly under the face of God. A poignant picture of unity, the worship reminded me that someday every people; every tribe, tongue and nation will join in the song of the Lamb. Many moments of sheer elation overwhelmed me while living onboard. I recognized this unspeakable joy as only a foretaste of the glory of heaven. Our lives in Canada had never known this kind of daily corporate worship.

It didn't take long for me to understand that worship is vital and central to the work and mission of Mercy Ships. It's part of the battle plan, a tool for spiritual warfare. Two lines from my favourite worship chorus (*We Will Dance* by David Ruis) celebrated the hope and the reason for our sacrifice aboard this vessel. Heaven.

> And we will dance on the streets that are golden,
> The glorious bride and the great Son of man...

Here on this earth, the streets are far from golden. The worn carpeted hallways of the Mercy Ship, the hard cobblestone streets of Europe and the dusty red earth of Africa had become our byways. Nevertheless, great energy, joy and healing flowed through the power and unity of worship onboard. It kept weary sailor missionaries walking the streets and battling the war against suffering, poverty, disease and spiritual degradation. Worship linked with our mission and work.

Mercy Ships is the world leader in delivering free health care to the world's forgotten poor. With the use of hospital ships carrying multi-national crew, world-class medical assistance and long-term sustainable development have been making a difference. Mercy Ships uses Jesus' model in Matthew 11:5: The *blind* see through cataract operations; the *lame* walk through orthopaedic surgeries; the *mute* speak through cleft-lip and palate operations; the walking *dead* are raised through life-saving maxillo-facial tumour operations; and the good news is preached through evangelism and teaching teams.

Many have asked, why ships? Most of the world's poor lives within 150 kilometres of a port city; most of these people do not have any access to medical care. I learned quickly that I had taken health care for granted in Canada. The majority of the world's population does not have access to a doctor, nurse, pharmacist, dentist or surgeon. The ramifications of this fact are colossal throughout our world! Soon I would witness the effects with my own eyes!

Ebb and Flow of Community Life

Boisterous chatter in the dining room, endless PA announcements, long queues at the snack bar and people strolling on Promenade Deck occurred as common daily events of community life. On B-deck, an area called Town Square comprising a post office, the PFO (Personal Finance Office) and hair salon became a gathering place as in any village.

Further aft, the laundry room with banks of washers and dryers, by virtue of necessity, remained a frequented hub. Crew signed for one-hour slots of washer and dryer time. To miss either of these slots meant either dirty clothes or wet laundry, therefore, laundry times tended to rule our lives.

Giving up personal rights, independence and the kind of freedom that westerners enjoy daily could sometimes prove to be the greatest challenge for a crewmember. For the health of the ship community, it proved absolutely vital. Exemplary crew members would pick up after themselves, wait patiently in line, think of others ahead of their own needs, diligently keep the many rules and work for the good of the community. Naturally, we fell short at times. In good humour, Captain Malcolm reminded crew that their mothers weren't there to pick up after them! Keeping the ship tidy seemed to be a never-ending battle.

Community life provided endless prime opportunities for God to reveal our selfish, prideful attitudes, and sometimes our inconsiderate and prejudicial natures. For example, how easily could I walk away graciously without displaying any indignation when an African day worker snatched the last coveted cinnamon bun? *He was not even a crewmember! Am I not more deserving than he?* My selfish thoughts demanded. *I paid crew fees and this ship was my home!*

Or as a homemaker of 14 years, how did I feel about having the captain do weekly cabin inspections of my home, my nest, and my territory? With difficulty, I laid down my homemaker rights and submitted to the required scrutiny. Good humouredly, he enjoyed ruffling my feathers and remarked about the tiniest fuzzes on my worn carpet.

How would I react to another parent or single crewmember correcting my child inappropriately? Rather than stewing inside or rising up like a mother bear, I needed to learn graciousness and sometimes put forth a loving presentation of my parental boundaries to others.

How should I respond to being awakened by late night conversations in the hallway outside our door? Sleep is crucial to my health and having it disturbed thoughtlessly irritated me. Most people responded apologetically as soon as I sleepily opened the cabin door. All was forgiven.

During our first few months onboard, I had become distraught and discouraged about our small cabin and began to pray earnestly for an upper deck cabin. The added space would allow us to eat meals together and enable more family activity within the cabin. When God answered my prayer several months later, I had no idea that it would come with a price tag.

Cabin selection was based on many factors besides seniority. Following a mass exodus of crew due to the heat and difficulties in Benin, upper deck family cabins began to open up. The housing selection committee followed a procedure to give optimum fairness before the offering of a cabin. To our delight, the offering of a lovely, large (relatively speaking) cabin fell to us—the exact one I had prayed for.

Herein we discovered one of the foremost areas for disunity to fester among crew members. Giving up rights to a comfortable nest hits nearly everyone at the heart. Unbeknownst to us, a few parents disgruntled by the selection procedure thought it unfair that we'd received Cabin 14. Simonne Dyer, the ship's CEO, called a meeting to discuss the issues, correct any misunderstandings and dispel hard feelings. Prior to this meeting, Bruce and I lived completely unaware that a storm brewed around us. To discover that we were the center of it shocked us at the meeting. I couldn't conceal my tears of pain. For the sake of unity, Bruce and

I considered giving up the coveted cabin to another family. But the decision remained unchanged. Time and forgiveness eventually healed the pain of that incident and we once again lived in harmony.

As expected, we faced many opportunities in our floating village to offer and receive forgiveness. Openness and loving confrontation was the policy I had always lived by when facing relational conflicts in the past. It proved highly successful over our four years with the Mercy Ship community. Other than a few knocks to my sensitive ego, my relationships remained healthy.

The challenges of the flesh became numerous when living so closely with brothers and sisters in Christ. Sometimes God pruned us in areas that touched the core of our natural human responses. At times I wondered if I could still love the one who repeatedly broke rules or occasionally stole another's possessions. Although the rare violation of theft incensed and saddened me the most, I learned to accept people at various levels of maturity and recognize my own propensity to sin in other areas. My respect for leadership grew as I observed how they handled these major violations. Showing great discretion, they focused their concern on the individual and their walk with Christ. Their example of discipline and accountability bestowed with mercy taught me to always strive for mercy over judgment.

Above all these challenges, how we delighted in the joy of true fellowship! I couldn't help but think that Jesus meant exactly this when encouraging his followers to dwell in unity. Like the New Testament Church, we lived together and experienced a true fellowship of the body of Christ.

A great forum for encouragement, venting, challenge, prayer and support happened in cell groups. Crowding weekly into each other's cabins, we treasured our fellowship with these special friends. Not only did we share emotional and spiritual closeness, our knees nearly touched each other in the smaller cabins. Our cell group increased our joy, connection, motivation and inspiration to carry on serving the King.

As we shifted through the two seasons of outreach in West Africa and the procurement phase in Europe, life with Mercy Ships altered greatly. For five to seven months, we remained docked in one port of West Africa, then for the rest of the year we sailed from port to port in Europe every three weeks. Our work changed dramatically in each phase. This cycle kept a heightened sense of purpose, adventure and excitement along with a constant ebb and flow of community life. It could be witnessed regularly in warm welcomes of newcomers, and tearful farewells of friends at the gangway.

Saying farewell seemed the most difficult aspect about living on the ship. Precious friends returned to their far corners of the earth, changing life onboard once again. Deep and abiding friendships sometimes faded into a mist of silent tears dropping to the ocean as we sailed away from the dock. This side of eternity, we met and shared a season of love, loyalty and common purpose. Then they were gone, awaiting a joyous reunion in heaven someday.

Long-term crew sometimes became reluctant to connect deeply with transient short-term people for this very reason. Often short-termers sensed this withholding and misunderstood the nature of its reality, but the heart can only withstand so much sorrow from constant separating.

Community life aboard Mercy Ships felt like a small foretaste of heaven. Rarely did we experience the kind of pettiness that so often ruins or divides churches in the West, nor the kind of fighting that occurs over theological issues. We rarely learned the religious denomination of our closest friends, because it was a non-issue. Our goal to serve the poor with the two hands of the gospel remained foremost and undeterred.

Because Jesus lives at the center of the Mercy Ships community, it bears a strong witness to the world—a floating village of love and mercy. With so much potential for disharmony arising from diversity, the greatest miracle was unity!

As a family, we treasured the time living in our floating village. For the rest of our lives, we will carry countless cherished memories—people laughing and praying together; people sweating and struggling; people serving and loving; mercy and generosity abounding. Bearing the hardships together, people became stronger as one.

However, we only reached this view of living in community through the perspective of time. For the first eight to twelve months after boarding, we faced four vital stages of adjustment: honeymoon, hostility, humour and homecoming.

19

The Homecoming

I am clay and I am water
Falling forward in this order
While the world spins 'round so fast
Slowly I'm becoming who I am

Nothing ever stays the same
The wheel will always turn
I feel the fire in the change
But somehow it doesn't burn
Like a beggar blessed I stumble in the Grace
Reaching out my hand for what awaits
Margaret Becker
Lyrics - Clay and Water

Honeymoon

 Swept up by the excitement of living our dream, we embraced our new community of faith and the joy of sailing to many countries with the message of hope and healing. We saw how the deep faith of the pioneers who began the mission continued to carry it through!

 Deeply touching times of prayer and unity often centered on a patient in distress down in the operating room or ICU. A public announcement of a medical emergency rallied people to prayer in their workplaces. Others stood outside the operating rooms, placing their hands on the walls as they cried for God to intervene for a patient's life. Many times we rejoiced at the raising of another life from the brink of death.

Death rarely touched our floating hospital and community. The low percentage of casualties, injuries and death onboard raised eyebrows amongst the shipping world. Experts concluded that we must have inaccurately recorded our numbers through the years since they were far too low for the average ship of that size and passenger volume, let alone for a hospital. If only they knew the power of prayer and unity to protect. This coupled with a diligence for safety by caring godly officers and engineers drove fear and calamity from us.

Calamity did, however, threaten and stare us in the face now and then! We discovered some of the hazards of ship life within a week after our arrival. One night, in youthful exuberance, Jillian jumped from the top bunk to her bed on the floor. On the flight downward, her long, chocolate-brown hair caught in the ceiling-mounted water sprinkler. Dangling by her hair, she swung momentarily. The boys screamed and we scurried into their room. We arrived seconds after she dropped to the floor. Distressed, the boys quickly blurted out the story as Jill lay in shock. Like some Indian scalp trophy, a wad of thick, long hair hung eerily from the sprinkler. A large coin-sized bald spot on her head prickled with tiny pores of blood. That night I tossed and turned, reliving the horror of it all.

Though shaken, we rejoiced when the crew hairstylist told us Jill's hair would grow in again. In the meantime, she parted her hair conveniently on that side. After sharing the story, we heard

Chapter Nineteen

many stories of family accidents upon arrival. Apparently families entering missions are a great source of irritation to the enemy of the Kingdom of God.

Despite this disturbing event, the honeymoon phase extended for several long blissful months. Bruce basked in the joy of teaching in his own classroom and the children happily settled into the exciting onboard school of 55 children. I tackled the challenge of my new position as deck secretary.

Our three young sailors delighted in the short jaunt down the hallway to their friends' cabins. Children's play converged at the ship jungle gym or playground area on aft deck where sufficient space allowed for a crowded game of floor hockey or basketball. The boys recovered numerous overboard balls and plastic pucks with a rope and basket device. Several floated away to small specks on the horizon as children watched helplessly. We accepted it as one of the perils of ship sports.

Hostility

With great resistance, our family slowly became distressed. The heat of tropical West Africa on a non air-conditioned ship proved to be unbearable. Virtually all crewmembers displayed heat rash on some part of their body. One fair-skinned man nicknamed 'Big Daddy' suffered with a nasty, angry rash all over his body. He attracted everyone's empathy as he forged through his daily welding tasks. Sweat dripped from our noses and down our backs while soggy desk papers stuck to our arms. People moved wearily about their duties taking random showers or standing directly in front of a fan to keep cool.

CEO Don Stephens, visiting the *Anastasis* in Benin, delivered a consoling message as he struggled with his damp shirt and wiped sweat from his brow. Addressing our difficult living conditions, he called them abusive to the body and determined to seek a way to obtain air-conditioning aboard the *Anastasis*. He admitted that it wouldn't be an easy task to raise funds for this kind of project.

I recall an incident where I seemed to lose the battle against heat. After a lukewarm shower (no cold water existed in the ship's pipes), I carefully dressed so as to avoid stirring up body heat. Within minutes, I felt suffocatingly hot and horrible. Standing directly in front of a floor fan, I strained for a measure of coolness while tears of anger and frustration released. "Are you ok, dear?" Bruce probed with pity in his eyes.

"I can't handle this anymore!" I answered angrily. I felt ashamed at my inability to cope with the conditions that day. Evening's slightly cooler temperatures brought no relief. The recommended solution to sleep easier? Wear a soaked T-shirt and let the fans blow directly over our bodies. That helped somewhat.

Bruce's new health condition raised concerns for the crew doctor. With his liver already compromised from Hepatitis C, should he take anti-malaria pills? Our doctor began to experiment, starting with the strongest pill, warning that should his body not tolerate them, he would be required to leave the ship. The threat alarmed us momentarily, but we soon forgot it in the daily grind of survival. Thankfully, he reacted no differently than most other crewmembers to the effects of anti-malarials.

A combination of heat and anti-malaria tablets kept many people awake at night. Sometimes during these sleepless nights, I wandered up on Promenade Deck for fresh air, only to find others quietly doing the same. To sleep fully through the night and awaken refreshed happened about one in four nights during our first outreach to West Africa.

Chapter Nineteen

As the honeymoon phase faded into the hostility phase, our children faced homesickness. Chadwick, who finds the change process most challenging, began to exhibit difficulties. Being an otherwise compliant, easy-going, delightful child, we recognized the problem as stemming from the enormous change we had undergone. We chose to set up a solid structure around him, with rules and consequences sticky-tacked to the cupboard door. Assuring him that we loved him too much to allow his life to fall apart, we applied strong measures that pulled him through this insecure time in his life. Before falling asleep at night, he placed a cardboard 'Shield of Faith' on his chest, which he'd crafted in Bible class at school. Three years later he could be heard saying he never wanted to leave the ship!

Jillian became highly emotional, prompting us to seek a change in her anti-malaria pills. A weaker dose gradually returned her to her normal self. The crew doctor had warned parents to watch for these side effects.

One night after flicking on the light, a flurry of insects mysteriously appeared and vanished. Checking the source, I discovered small mounds of tiny eggs on the wooden ledge by Chad's bunk. Inside the light fixture, a dead sample of this invasion confirmed my suspicion. Termites. We lived just above the carpentry deck where lumber is stored. Apparently that very cabin had been fumigated for the same problem years before. The captain agreed to seal the fate of these creatures promptly. For several nights, the children dispersed to different sleeping quarters. Even after spraying, they needed coaxing to relieve their fears about termites in our cabin.

Although our cabin provided a refuge, the confined space meant that our children spent more time away from it.

Understandably, they met and played for hours with friends on aft deck or in the ship pool. As a result, our family unit slowly crumbled. Former family routines that lent stability no longer existed. Our tiny cabin didn't allow room to eat meals together. Dispersed into community, it seemed we'd lost our sense of family. Something needed to change.

One night after comforting one of our crying children from missing their family and friends, Bruce turned to me in exasperation, "Is all this worth it?" The confined spaces, the insomnia, the stress of the heat and anti-malaria pills on our bodies, the pain our children experienced…it all felt like too great a sacrifice. At this stage, the temptation to leave grew stronger than ever.

Many short-term missionaries due to the shorter length of service never move beyond the honeymoon stage to enter this difficult phase of adjustment to their new surroundings. Perseverance and focusing on the purpose of our calling seemed to be the key for us.

Had we not already walked through the Potter's fires in preparation for this time, I doubt whether we could have moved past this stage and remained onboard. Understandably, some people did not. The sheer fact of an aging ship demanding constant repairs could cause any saint to throw their hands up in exasperation. For others, the spiritual battles proved too tiring.

Our post-war generation, having been raised in relative ease and comfort is sometimes unprepared for the challenges and discomforts of missionary living. When life gets tough, we seek ways of releasing ourselves immediately from the struggle for more comfortable options. Perseverance and longsuffering are not high on the list of virtues sought after by our generation. We are highly committed to our ease, satisfaction and well-being. Too quickly, we abandon situations causing us pain. I observed that the African people bear up far more patiently than Westerners under adverse conditions. For them, struggle and perseverance are a lifestyle. We have much to learn from a nation where the human spirit is stretched and strengthened against unbearable odds.

Decidedly, for the sake of the poor and just one African life changed for eternity, Bruce and I agreed that all our struggles were worthwhile. Daily we witnessed lives transformed in the ward. Besides, we had given a verbal commitment of two years and would not renege on our word.

Humour

In the course of a year's time, the hostility phase fizzled to the humour phase. Together we learned to laugh about the cockroaches that pestered and unsettled us in our cabins and various parts of the ship. The largest variety of cockroaches acquired the nickname "Kona Kruisers" since they apparently first stowed aboard when the ship docked in Kona, Hawaii. We shared funny stories of how best to kill them. Bruce often experienced the strange tickle of a cockroach crawling up his leg from the shower drain. Some people learned to wash their hair with eyes opened to watch for the critters. It all made humorous dining room conversations.

Hassles of living without water for hours on end and having flushing turned off regularly for sewage treatment repairs were gradually taken in stride and bantered about lightly. Playing practical jokes on others and howling at skits about culturally insensitive missionaries became part of the mirth we came to know onboard.

As the saying goes, 'when life hands you lemons, make lemonade', our boys decidedly made some of their own. Fans in the portholes sucked in the dusty air of the Harmattan desert winds, leaving a brown film on furniture and cupboards. Mosquito nets over the portholes quickly became coated with the dust, blocking out the light. Despite this, I always welcomed the Harmattan because the sand-filled winds also blocked the penetrating equatorial sun and afforded somewhat cooler temperatures. Keeping nets dusted and fans cleaned meant a brighter and cleaner cabin. Showing entrepreneurial spirit, our boys took advantage of the dusty fan problem onboard. A fan cleaning business proved to be a lucrative venture for them. Their notices around the ship read:

> FAN CLEANING!
> Brandon and Chadwick's
> Spick and Span Fan Company.

At 75 cents per fan, they unscrewed blades, washed and shone them up, then returned them spotless and gleaming to their owners. Our shower floor sometimes bore the evidence of that grimy undertaking, after which I threatened to take a cut of the profits! This seemed to do the trick without deterring their entrepreneurial spirit. The floors stayed cleaner after that.

Gradually, the nuisances and inconveniences of ship life were overlooked and sprinkled with humour. Little by little, we flexed and stretched and laughed together.

Homecoming

A Swiss crewmember offered a free flat in Switzerland for our first vacation taken off the ship. Mountains, wide open spaces,

Chapter Nineteen   Page 151

and the awesome feeling of freedom welcomed us. After all the adjustments of living onboard, it felt like a breath of fresh air. In the tiny village of Morël, nestled deep in the Alps, we found solitude and refreshment. Opening the shutters of our Swiss holiday flat each morning, fresh mountain breezes drifted through our window.

Aside from hiking mountain trails and playing in clear, glacial streams, we planned to review and evaluate our family life as missionaries. Praying for wisdom, we explored ways to better preserve our family unit and ensure healthy living onboard. Through our discussions, we began to draw up new rules and systems. We arranged a schedule for the children's homework times, exclusive family and movie nights, daily meals in the cabin, and family devotions. Then we set rules about friends in the cabin and communicating whereabouts. I designed a laminated sign for our cabin door that would give opportunity for friends to post messages when we were unavailable during our family times. These simple actions provided wonderful times of family privacy while living within a bustling community. Like a sports team needing time-out for a huddle, our family needed to regularly re-group to encourage and cheer one another.

For most crewmembers, finding places of peaceful solitude in our community home required creativity. Since Bruce's brother had sent us tins of flavored coffee for Christmas, we agreed to find a special time and place to enjoy it together. As a result, our weekly tradition of sharing hazelnut and amaretto coffee began. Depending on the season and hemisphere, we found either a corner in the Med Lounge or a table out on Promenade Deck. Our early Saturday morning "coffee date" grew to be a delightful time that we anticipated each week. While the children slept or played Lego not far away, we shared the joy of companionship in those relaxed conversations together as husband and wife.

Settling into the homecoming stage is marked by flexibility as well as acceptance of annoyances and hardships. Together we adapted and accepted all that came with our new way of life. Moving to the larger coveted cabin of 375 square feet, along with a new air conditioning system installed in our third year also did wonders to transform our living experience while in West Africa.

Our new family plans for ship living proved the most successful. Almost immediately we experienced the benefits of the changes we'd made following our review in Switzerland. From that time onward, ship life moved from bearable to wonderful. Surprisingly, after this first return to the *Anastasis*, we realized that it truly felt like we had come home! Indeed serving God aboard a hospital ship would be possible after all.

20
Weeping with the Wounded

> *And if you spend yourselves in behalf of the hungry and satisfy the needs of the oppressed, then your light will rise in the darkness, and your night will become like the noonday.*
> *Isaiah 58:10*

The colour of the sea changed from deep ocean blues to aqua greens and then to murky brown yellows near the coast. The word spread quickly throughout the ship. Africa was finally in sight once again!

The familiar scent of Africa wafted across the waves, triggering a plethora of memories from our previous visit—a strong mixture of fish and cooking fires magnified by the humidity. I recalled the pungent scents of earthy fruits and vegetables, dried fish and goat heads in the marketplaces.

A TV camera or National Geographic photos can never truly capture and convey Africa. One needs to experience the full bodied scents and sounds that accompany this vast, magnificent continent.

The familiar sounds gradually reached us from the shores of Conakry, Guinea. How I loved the splendid beat of African goat-skinned drums! As we drew closer, I recognized the distant thunder of dilapidated cars, motor bikes and heavy diesel trucks on crowded city streets, bearing few traffic lights or road rules. I recollected the haunting calls of beggars as they crawled on hands and knees.

Soon we would taste the sweetness of plantain, fresh pineapples and mangoes, coconut and ground nuts. We would again need to be wary of African food preparation, taking precautionary measures for our delicate Western digestive system.

Fishing villages marked by tin-roofed huts dotted the shoreline. My thoughts turned to the women of Africa—women who work harder than any other people in the world. Dwarfed by the bulk of the oncoming Mercy Ship, the African men drifted out to sea in worn fishing canoes. It might be days before they returned.

From the rails of Promenade Deck, we sighted dark, shiny faces in the blazing sun. Wearing bright clothing of varied texture, colour and design, the African people stood in the forefront of this magnificent scenery of green palm trees and sandy shores. Huge banners of welcome greeted us from the dock.

A church choir clad in satiny, turquoise robes lined the cement pier. With rhythmical movement, their bodies swayed and danced to tunes of praise and worship. Abruptly, 26 policemen and numerous soldiers arrived, placing themselves strategically along the dock as a strong show of the promised security. It seemed a daunting contrast of rhythmical worship and hardened military strength. It revealed a picture of two kinds of warfare, one for flesh and blood and one for the unseen world of principalities and powers.

A band carrying dented, dingy instruments marched in celebration. Pockets of women in the crowd danced freely, African style. Hips swaying and arms moving in perfect rhythm, they waved white handkerchiefs in celebration. These are the greetings of a culture so different from our own.

Chapter Twenty

While celebrations continued, mooring operations proceeded to manoeuvre the ship into our berth, our new location for the next five months. Our new CEO, Dr. Gary Parker, made his way down the gangway, setting his feet firmly on African soil after a two week journey on the seas. Formalities, speeches and ceremonies commenced on the dock while we watched from the rails.

Members from our Mercy Ship's Advance Team joined in these events on the dock, their white faces easy to spot. Boarding the ship, they reunited with their Mercy Ship family. In preparation for the ship's visit, they'd been selected and commissioned to precede the ship five months prior to our arrival. Working with government officials, agencies, existing medical structures, churches, missionaries and more, they prearranged our work. The advance team selected land sites for our mobile medical and dental services, hired translators, initiated security measures, and secured water and fuel sources all before our arrival.

Before given permission to go ashore, crew attended a mandatory orientation. Advance Team members informed us about the customs and history of the country, its people groups as well as the current political and spiritual climate. They offered practical tidbits of information ranging from local churches to attend and locations of markets to the names of con men to avoid. They also warned about cultural insensitivities that could harm our expression of Christ.

I regarded this orientation meeting as essential for both new and old missionaries seeking to navigate their way in a foreign culture. The arrival of 400 Christians converging on one country is an enormous threat to the spiritual realms of darkness. The devil, our true enemy, seeks ways to devour us, to con and steal from us and to send us away from his strongholds of despair and hopelessness that grip the nation.

Therefore, I deemed it wise to heed the information from those who like Joshua's returning spies had already scoped out the territory. I saw the importance of hearkening to the words about the giants in the land, without feeling intimidated. Armed with this knowledge and strengthened in unity, we could be *as wise as serpents and harmless as doves* in staking the nation for the Kingdom of God. Sometimes our strong presence alone in African nations penetrated the darkness and brought obvious transformation to both physical and spiritual realms.

Customs officers soon embarked to begin the long process of stamping hundreds of passports. Hours later, an overhead announcement declared the ship cleared. With shouts and cheers, we finally stepped on land—released to bring mercy to Africa, to offer hope and healing to the poor.

I remember the first time our family set foot on African soil. We walked out of the port thrilled with the wonder of it all. Like David Livingstone, Mary Slessor and scores of missionaries before us, we had sailed into Africa for the purpose of sharing the gospel. What a privilege to be a part of this same great commission!

The mission began once customs released our cargo and vehicles. A fleet of Mercy Ship Land Rovers could be seen heading out of the port each morning. Teams of dental workers, community health teachers, doctors, construction workers, water and sanitation workers, counsellors, evangelists, puppeteers and musicians left eagerly to affect sustainable change for the poor.

In the early stages of our life in Africa, I often felt perplexed over how an entire continent managed to progress so slowly. Some of our first impressions felt like we had time-warped back to Bible days. Unfamiliar customs, long flowing robes, and dusty roads seemed to set us back a few thousand years. While the rest of the world seemed to be spinning changes faster than a spider's webs, why did Africa seem so far behind? What caused such stagnancy? We would never understand completely, but our eyes would be opened along the way.

Screening Days

With an added bounce of excitement in his step, Brandon pranced down for breakfast in the Pacific Dining Room. He poured himself the usual glass of shelf preserved milk and a heaping bowl of cereal. His classmates Mathias and Joel joined him at the breakfast table.

Today would be different from the routine of ordinary classes. A few days after the ship's arrival to coastal West Africa, screening days for surgery appointments began at the local stadium. Brandon and his peers would spend the day at the screening site helping where needed. Today they would share in the venture as vessels of mercy to the poor.

I caught a later vehicle shuttle to join Brandon at the site. Although still early morning, already the heat penetrated my ship uniform—a white cotton shirt with shoulder bars, marine epaulettes and a black skirt. I wondered how I would last the day. At physically demanding times such as these, I became fully aware of my health limitations, but determined to work beyond them by leaning on the grace of God. I kept my water bottle close at hand.

As we drove the dusty streets, I prayed for strength and thought of the many Africans who endured physical suffering far greater than my own. Many of them would have heard about the ship's arrival by radio, posters or word of mouth. A medical screening being held at the stadium had been announced throughout the country. From the north, people travelled by taxi for days. Some pooled all their money to afford the trip. Most of them had exhausted every effort with local doctors, witch doctors, herbs and medicines to find healing, but still they suffered. For many, Mercy Ships was their last hope. A foreign doctor offering free surgery could be their last chance for survival.

When the Land Rover bearing the Mercy Ships name and logo slowly passed through throngs of people at the gates to the stadium, heads turned curiously to stare at us. Imploring eyes questioned, "Are you the doctors that can help me?" I could scarcely believe the magnitude of the crowd, estimated at over 3,000. Queues of Africans, in multicoloured clothing, wove passively around the stadium. The crowds resembled my grandmother's braided mats of colourful design created from remnants of fabric.

There appeared to be peace and order at the hands of the local police and Mercy Ship volunteers. Previous experience with the desperate crowds of West Africa's poor had taught us to be aware of the potential for rioting and chaos. One of the best weapons for this kind of crisis is prayer. Volunteer prayer warriors from the crew discreetly surrounded the crowds, while back at the *Anastasis* a prayer vigil took place in the ship's lounge. Partners from home countries around the world joined in prayer for these two days.

No matter how often I faced these needy crowds, nothing quite prepared my heart for the reality of poverty and suffering *en masse*. For up to two days, they waited patiently in the hot sun with little access to food and water. Some had to be turned away because of terminal illness with cancer, or an inoperable problem. Escorted to the prayer station, we shared the love of Jesus and prayed for them.

Miracles were not unheard of at these prayer stations. One

Chapter Twenty

man blinded by disease felt his eyes water when a crewmember prayed for his healing. Suddenly daylight pierced through to his sensitive eyes. Someone ran for sunglasses and the man returned home rejoicing, no longer needing surgery.

I hold an image of Brandon that day that will forever stir my heart. He and his classmates served a host of blind people waiting at the eye station. They gave a cup of cold water in the name of Jesus to thirsty, grateful people. But wrenching questions glared and churned in my soul. Why had my son been born in a wealthy country where hot and cold water runs freely? A place where people can fill swimming pools without a second thought? Will Brandon always remember the poor he helped this day?

Still other questions arose while I carried out my tasks. Why do I have lifelong access to medication for my thyroid disease when these women must shamefully hide their profuse goitres under scarves around their neck? Thyroid pills are unavailable or unaffordable to them. *Why am I so blessed?*

After escorting the blind and those with tumours and cleft lips to the appropriate stations, I met a young crewmember quietly sobbing as she walked to gather more people. I understood. We both wept for the pain of the people. Somehow we choked back the tears and carried on. "Did Jesus weep when he healed the multitudes?" I asked myself.

During one screening process, I found myself at the intake station. With the help of a translator I recorded medical histories for maxillo-facial (tumours, cleft lip and palate) patients. These men, women and children had already been screened and selected for surgery by our staff. Now they waited in a new line, eyes filled with hope.

Surprising to me, many of the people had no clue about their age, especially the older women. How could anyone not know his or her age? My translator simply guessed at the year of their birth. This bewildered me. Are there no birthday parties to mark the years in this culture? No cake or presents, no streamers and birthday hats? Somehow in the heat and pain of this screening process, that all seemed laughable and silly—customs from some trite place.

I watched Dr. Gary Parker, our Chief Medical Officer, as he examined patients. He probed and prodded gently around the tumour and then smiled at the patient. Gary's expression of love and compassion was worth a thousand words to the suffering one not understanding English. Dr. Gary became 'Jesus with skin on' to them. Through a translator, hope sprang anew within the heart of the deformed, disfigured individual. Blood work and an identification photo snapped for the file completed the screening process. An appointment card in hand meant the ticket to life-changing surgery.

At the end of the day, I returned to the ship feeling like a clay vessel utterly poured out. In the solitude of our cabin, I flopped into a chair. Then it came unexpectedly. The bottled up tears of the day flowed freely to my lap. Images kept drifting through my brain and piercing my heart. Images of tumours the size of cantaloupes protruding from faces, blind people groping along, flesh eaten away by disease, ropes of skin and tissue distorting lovely faces, burns and scars, goitres and crippled children… thousands of them.

I had seen enough poverty and disease to unsettle me for a lifetime. How could my life ever be the same?

21

Hope and Healing

The blind receive sight, the lame walk, those who have leprosy are cured, the deaf hear, the dead are raised, and the good news is preached to the poor.

Matthew. 11:5

When I encountered Mutala coming down the steps accompanied by a nurse, an awkward moment followed. I withheld the gasp, but he had sensed my shock as his one eye met mine. I recovered and smiled, conveying my acceptance and love. He seemed to respond, but it was obvious that he knew the impact his disfigurement had on people.

Parents had taken a knife to the tumour growing from three-year-old Mutala's head. But no amount of cutting or squeezing could remove the lump. A witch doctor told them if they tried to remove it, he would die. At age 16, the 14-inch neurofibroma tumour drooped heavily and swung with the movement of his body like a football in a netted sack. His right eye had become misshapen and stretched down near his chin level. His appearance reminded me of wax crayons that had sat too long in the back window of a car on a hot day. Little wonder he kept his face wrapped up and rarely ventured into public. I'd grown accustomed to seeing hideous tumours and disfigurement, but his face was beyond painful to look upon. This young man needed a miracle.

When Mutala Drammeh arrived in the ward, he promptly hid his face in the blankets. Ward nurses sitting inches from his bed prayed that God would protect his life, guide the surgeons during the surgery and reveal His love for Mutala during the recovery time.

But Mutala came to us at an inconvenient time. Surgery schedules were already booked solid for the remainder of our stay in The Gambia. Weary medical staff and surgeons anticipated a restful renewal over the Easter holiday weekend ahead. But who could ever turn away this man? Who could refuse mercy to such a soul? We are MERCY Ships. And this man had great need of mercy.

The painful, frightening ordeal ended in the death of a huge, disfiguring tumour. It happened on Good Friday. The young man's subsequent resurrection from the grave of rejection, humiliation and isolation lay ahead. The operation performed by Dr. Gary Parker and Dr. Ian McColl, a general surgeon from Britain, took 12 intense hours and required 16 "*Anastasis* units" of blood. They were unable to remove the entire tumour, nor to salvage his left ear or eye. A further surgery would be required on our subsequent visit two years later. For now, the bulk of the mass had been severed and Mutala's life saved. He recovered remarkably well.

He would likely never realize the many sacrifices that contributed to his successful surgery that Good Friday. Staff in the operating room had worked overtime on a holiday weekend while their children missed them; crewmembers remained onboard to give blood. Indirectly others had sacrificed for Mutala, including various corporations who donated equipment and supplies, and donors who gave faithfully to the work. This act of mercy demonstrated the unrelenting love of God for a shy, reclusive African teenager. Many people, many sacrifices, but no sacrifice would equal the one made by Jesus 2000 years before on a cross.

Hands of Thanksgiving

Bruce and the children will never forget meeting Malick Bogumo. During chapel period, he visited their school on A-deck and spoke to the students. He seemed to understand the sacrifice the children had made so their parents could serve with Mercy Ships. While holding their hands, he warmly thanked them for being there. Malick acknowledged that their willingness to follow their parents had given him a life-saving surgery.

Naturally a patient would think to express gratitude to the director of the ship, or surgeons, nurses and even ordinary crewmembers. To have the understanding and insight to consider and thank the least of those among us, the children, seemed outstanding. Our children enjoyed a quiet moment of honour and gratitude for all the sacrifices they'd made to be missionary kids; sacrifices they'd long forgotten in the joy of living aboard this wonderful Mercy Ship.

Following his moving speech, he displayed some of his woven handbags, a business that supported his wife and family. Despite the 3.05-kg. tumour on his jaw, (the heaviest removed in Mercy Ships history) Malick had not let it overcome his life. Though people treated him differently because of the abnormality, he chose to interact socially as normally as possible. His energetic, outgoing personality had won friends, but he always wondered how long it would be before the tumour finally took his life. In 1987 he had become a Christian and nine years later, he married. His wife had told him matter-of-factly that she would never become a Christian unless God removed that tumour.

Hearing of the upcoming visit of the Mercy Ship through local missionaries in a nearby village, Malick began to hope for the first time in 40 years. He joined with others needing the help of Mercy Ships and journeyed to the coastal city of Conakry.

Three months following successful surgeries, Malick headed home to his village of Lola, set in the shadow of Nimbia Mountain of south eastern Guinea. Imagine his anticipation in showing his wife and village his new appearance. His daughter Marie took several days to adjust to this new daddy without the plaguing tumour. His wife, Maciami, could hardly believe her eyes, nor could she ignore what God had done for him. She received his God as her Saviour.

Two weeks later the activities of Lola village came to a halt for a great celebration. Butchering two sheep and four chickens for the feast, villagers and neighbours danced and paraded through the dusty streets to celebrate Malick's successful surgery. Everyone wore t-shirts emblazoned with a hand pointing up. Below the hand it read, "Thanks be to God." Hands, hands, hands everywhere in the crowd pointed upward. Hands of thanksgiving gave glory where glory was due.

Malick returned to the ship for one final surgery to remove the last flap of excess skin from his cheek. He received a homecoming welcome from the crew and could often be heard saying, "Thanks be to God for renewing my life through the people of the *Anastasis*."

Kernel of Wheat

Success stories seemed the norm of our encounters onboard. Sometimes my faith rested more in the miracle hands of our surgeons and nurses than in the hands of the Great Physician.

Chapter Twenty One

Rare patients like Cavilla drew me back to the reality of who held the keys to healing, to life and to death. Cavilla's experience is not the success story we'd come to expect. However, from an eternal perspective, her story looks entirely different.

A cancerous tumour the size of an orange protruded from Cavilla's eye. At the age of three, she was dying of Burkitt's disease. Sending out a worldwide plea for chemotherapy drugs to save her life, a US drug company responded. Cavilla and her parents began to hope. Treatments started and the aggressive cancer receded slowly, making it possible for our surgeons to operate on the remaining tumour.

Nurses and crew visiting the ward did everything to win the feisty three-year-old's affections, but she never learned to disassociate pain from the Yovo (white person). Following successful surgery, Cavilla began to have neurological problems: vomiting, slurred speech, seizures and periods of unconsciousness. All day the medical team agonized trying to determine the cause. The ship's crew took up her cause by praying earnestly while medical staff laboured through the night to save her life. But she slipped away. A deep mourning swept over the ship as everyone struggled with the news about the little one who had captured our hearts over the months.

With her lifeless body, nurses travelled in silence to her village. Uncharacteristic for his culture, the father met them and carried her body to his home, weeping loudly. During the funeral, Cavilla's father challenged the elders in the village to consider their lack of love and response to his child's need. Many had advised them to stop feeding her and leave her in a corner to die, to go on and have more children. He contrasted this with the extreme love and care shown her by the Mercy Ships people. With passion, he urged them to consider the God of the Christian *Yovo*."

Days later, the highest chiefs and elders of the village requested a visit to the ship. As is customary hospitality with all our guests, they embarked on a tour of the vessel. While being led to the bridge, a pinnacle of the tour, showing how the ship is steered, the chief commented, "This is all very nice, but we really want to know how to follow 'your Jesus way'."

After being given a hearty meal in the guest dining room, and a gospel message now so familiar to them, they all agreed that the time had come to follow Jesus. A pastoral counsellor led them in prayer. Serious about their conversion, they requested Bibles and someone to teach them. Most of their questions could be summed up in one statement, "How should we live now?"

In many African cultures, elders and chiefs are respected for their wisdom and maturity. Unlike our cultures where productivity is strongly esteemed and the voice of the aged is weak, Africa's elderly grow into a place of honour. Their decisions are heeded in their village communities. When the elders of Cavilla's village pondered and decided to follow "the Jesus way", the village revered that decision and many genuinely responded. It is similar to families of Jewish households in Jesus' day.

A weekly Bible study from a local missionary began for the entire village. Plans for a church were soon underway.

Like a single kernel of wheat falling to the ground, three year old Cavilla died. But a village lives eternally.

> Unless a kernel of wheat falls to the ground and dies, it remains only a single seed. But if it dies it produces many seeds.
> John 12:4

22

Clay Vessels of Mercy

Those who go down to the sea in ships...They have seen the works of the Lord, and His wonders in the deep.
Psalm 107:23 NASB

Because Mercy Ships uses ocean-going vessels to be instruments of God's mercy to the poor, often these ships are suitably termed 'vessels of mercy'. But the people who live and serve aboard them are also God's vessels of mercy—clay vessels in the hands of a Potter.

Our family's earlier years of personal hardship had burned compassion deep into the core of these clay vessels. It would come to be poured out as healing mercy to those living in far poorer circumstances and experiencing sufferings far greater than our own. As God restored hope and healing into our wounded spirits, we in turn could offer hope and healing to those in more desperate need.

As we settled into our fulfilling missionary life onboard, we reflected on the years of struggle at home. To say that we trusted in our loving God no longer seemed a flippant phrase uttered in religious sounding tones, but rather we offered it with conviction and the high cost of God's training in our lives. Through the fires, His divine love had touched us.

Because our Heavenly Father is the only worthy object of our complete trust, we had come to believe that all things in our lives would work out for our highest good. Admittedly what I feared most was that His highest good would mean further suffering or perhaps even tragedy in our lives. I had to surrender to this possibility and fully trust. As missionaries facing the unknown, we could embrace this loving God, abandoning ourselves to Him rather than fearing what lay around the corner.

Oswald Chambers speaks of this attitude of abandonment to His purposes.

> If God has made your cup sweet, drink it with grace; or even if He has made it bitter, drink it in communion with Him. If the providential will of God means a hard and difficult time for you, go through it...God is working in us to reach His highest goals until His purpose and our purpose become one.[1]

Trusting God is the foundational principle for living this Christian life and often when tested the strength of that trust is revealed. Bruce and I had agreed and understood that the long and difficult preparation years had served to strengthen our foundation of trust, to build our character and to prepare us as vessels of mercy serving with Mercy Ships.

The initial setback of Bruce's Hepatitis C did not hinder his work onboard. In time he put on weight, appearing and feeling healthy and energetic. Often we forgot that he carried a life-long disease while he served. Few people knew. For exercise, greatly needed while living on a ship, he gradually returned to his passion of biking.

In the country of The Gambia, paved roads and respect for laws lent themselves to better biking conditions than other West

Chapter Twenty Two

African nations. Bruce and two fellow West African crewmembers began to train together in the wee hours of the morning for a bike race. The exciting day for the 35-kilometer Gambian national race finally arrived. In the hazy heat of the African sun, Bruce's muscular legs carried his body with all the strength he could muster. I couldn't help but reflect on how he had persevered in the race of life that the Apostle Paul talks about in his letter to the Philippians.

At the end of the race, the children and I waited anxiously for Bruce to arrive. Like white dots, we stood out in the full stadium of dark-skinned Africans. Crowds cheered the winner enthusiastically as he rounded the corner, entered the stadium gates and raced into the inner track. Another great cheer rose when a toubob (white man) wheeled into fourth place ahead of the pack. From high in the stands, his family also cheered him in! For this 41-year-old white racer, it symbolized a victory of huge proportions. Only three years after a health crisis, God had restored, healed and allowed him to prosper in great health. He had been granted the joy of serving in missions to the fullest.

He considered his teaching career in the floating school a dream gift beyond his imagination. "I've got the best job on the ship," he often exclaimed. The delightful, fulfilling years onboard also afforded an emotional healing time from the struggles of the past. He regarded it a privilege to teach the children of dedicated, hard working missionaries: officers, plumbers, doctors, evangelists, carpenters, cooks, administrators, welders, journalists, surgeons, nurses and more. Alongside their parents, these children had been sent to the nations to serve and sacrifice. Their lives were unique, requiring care, teaching and nurturing.

In a snug classroom, his bold strong voice could be heard

above the day workers chipping paint and welders fixing steel. It competed with passing sea traffic, linesmen shouting orders for mooring operations, and the noisy ship propellers directly below the school.

To his students, their travelling classroom availed a varied and colourful hands-on education. Holland granted free tours of the Anne Frank Museum; the Republic of The Gambia offered the "Roots" tour (from Alex Haley's book) in a remote village. The students hiked the fjords of Norway and roving game parks of South Africa. They visited a classroom of Norwegian students and an orphanage of Benin's abandoned children.

Bruce's continual quests for playing fields for Physical Education class from port to port accented this educational field trip of the globe. This teacher taught with outdated computers and cramped spaces but he also taught with the unlimited resources of the world. He prepared lessons for high school English literature, math, science, Bible and Physical Education. And with great freedom he taught all truth built on the foundation of God's truth.

As students left the ship or graduated, they registered in universities and colleges around the world. A strong encouragement to the school came with the frequent word of students who had left the ship and were now scoring far above their peers. Younger students often proved to be a grade ahead in their home countries. Their unique cross cultural education coupled with the experience of community living well-equipped them for further education, and for life.

As our British principal, Sandy Burnett believed, "The children may have given up an awful lot in their home countries, but they've gained far more here onboard." Our own children heartily agree.

Chapter Twenty Two

For 10 years prior to living on the ship, my life had been devoted mainly to the raising of our children. Withdrawn from the work force, I had taught myself how to cope daily with the invisible disability of my thyroid condition and symptoms of chronic fatigue.

With the children happily engaged in school onboard, I could devote six hours of my day to my assigned job, that of deck secretary for the captain and officers. Still I remained anxious about juggling these two responsibilities and keeping my health stable. Learning the ropes around the deck and navigating uncharted waters of balancing work and parenting seemed high waves initially for this mother of three. Eventually the rhythm of ship life with its prepared meals and self-contained amenities proved desirable for my health condition.

As the aging Mercy Ship required upgrading to the new International Safety Maritime Organization (ISMO) standards and laws of safety, deadlines faced the captain and officers. Using the best of my organizational skills, I arranged the myriad of paper work into new orderly systems. A year and a half later, having passed the safety tests and reached our many goals, maintenance of the deck office remained my only challenge. The challenge soon faded into boredom. The isolation of Lido deck and lack of connection with other moms (or any females) eventually took their toll.

Months slipped by, leaving me feeling unfulfilled and unconnected to the ministry. In prayer, I asked God for a change and then turned to the Human Resources department for a new position. As I waited I asked God to avail this seemingly unproductive time as a "sponge time", where I could draw nearer to Him and soak up all that He had for me to learn. I then found myself in a process of separating my identity from my performance. This difficult separation would hopefully build a stronger foundation resting on my true identity in Christ, rather than on my productivity. I was learning to *be*, rather than *do*, and still consider myself valuable. Hidden in the shadows, it seemed that I had lost all confidence and previous identity from my life back in Canada. Believing that God was carrying out a hidden work in me brought me through those days. As I waited it out, the roots of abiding in Christ grew deeper.

Finally a change of course counteracted the winds of boredom and isolation. A new port of call in Port Elizabeth, South Africa heralded the beginning of change for me. Near the hospital wing on B deck, an old wooden deck leading to the medical administrator's office generated a whole new view, and a whole new action.

Africa's poor ambled these corridors, eyes filled with fear and hope at the prospect of surgery. Eyes filled with wonder—wonder at the sight of a floating hospital of steel and wood. To them it seemed a palace!

Wealthy Europeans and South Africans also walked these corridors marked by tour ropes. Their eyes also reflected amazement—their hearts moved by photo images of suffering and compassion. However, their wonder lay in the sight of so crude and cramped a home chosen by professionals to carry out their heroic service.

During the public relations phase in Europe, my new position as the medical administrator's assistant meant hours of preparation, organization, prayer and inspiration for two medical receptions, held in each new port. We prayed that God would move the wealthy medical communities beyond their comfortable lifestyles to give, to pray and go with us to the poor. Many responded.

During the outreach phase in Africa, my mission changed. Besides assisting with administrative responsibilities, my boss released me to seize endless opportunities with staff and patients. Administrative duties found me skirting through the hospital ward daily. Not being a medical person, at first the degree of suffering upset me and I found myself asking why we had to put these people through this. Slowly I grew to accept it as a place of suffering in order to bring healing. I realized then that often God treats us similarly. He uses circumstances that feel akin to major surgery in order to heal problems in our lives. Although the suffering feels horrendous at the time, healing and joy follow.

As I reflected upon my own personal suffering, mild by comparison, I remembered that it had produced a sense of unworthiness, yet I had grown up knowing this God of love. As I thought about the suffering of the poor in Africa, how much greater the rejection they must feel at the hands of an unknown Being. So many living with horrible tumours or cleft lip and palate disease already feel the rejection by their communities, who believe they are cursed by the gods.

I began to understand the depth of spiritual and physical transformation in patients' lives when they received Christ's love. To encounter such a patient prior to surgery and to see the same person weeks or months later is like encountering two different people in the same body. Before-and-after photos only capture part of that transformation. The miracle is to sense the spirit of the one so changed.

Times of celebration, worship and dancing often broke out in the ward. In this place of suffering and healing, I witnessed a blind man embracing a new world in living color, a new face for the outcast, and a new chubby grin for the formerly starving infant. Even more thrilling, I saw the light reflected in the eyes of all that had received the love of the Master. Many watched *The Jesus Film* in their own language several times over. The compelling love of that message combined with the care of nurses and doctors, crew visitors and Bible counsellors wooed many hearts to Him. In a nation where pure survival is the goal, compassionate action is rare. Many had never experienced anything like it before!

Transformed by a surgeon's hands on the outside, and transformed by Jesus' love on the inside—one by one, these miracles of hope filled my life. How I thanked God for granting our ordinary family the extraordinary privilege of being part of such noble work. Undeserving, possessing no great skills, and often operating in weakness, He chose to find us useful as clay vessels of mercy, sent to the poor.

The time came for our last day of outreach in West Africa before heading north. Days before, the ward began to shut down. Nurses dismantled beds and moved them aside in preparation for sailing to Europe. It didn't seem possible that the chatter of foreign tongues, clapping of tiny hands, clanging and banging, coughing and snoring had ceased. The ward had become a cavernous room in need of a deep cleaning. Doors to the empty operating rooms stood wide open. I entered freely crossing the taped red line without having to wear scrubs. There too, I paused and felt the empty, hollow ache. I had become strongly attached to the people and work of this fantastic floating hospital!

23

Cabin to Compound

Religion that God our Father accepts as pure and faultless is this: to look after orphans and widows in their distress...

James 1:27

From the moment they stepped in the door, I felt awkward and uneasy. Our tiny family cabin seen through Isatou's scanning eyes, suddenly felt exceedingly rich. The lovely pine roll-top desk donated by a Norwegian manufacturer must have seemed exquisite.

Having met Samba and his wife Isatou in the ward, we invited our African friends for a visit to our cabin. I'd enjoyed pleasant communication with Samba while his son Mafugi recovered from cleft lip and palate surgery. As a teacher in The Republic of The Gambia, he could speak fluent English. His wife understood very little and often requested translation in her tribal tongue.

As they sat on our soft couch, Isatou's eyes continually scanned about the room. While we carried on conversation with Samba, I noted her intrigue at the Monet print and the wooden framed photos of our children on the walls. A vase of flaming red silk tulips (from Holland of course) splashed color into our co-ordinates of blue and beige. The room carpeted in the dying remains of a once plush blue rug—at which I'd scowled inwardly during unsuccessful cleaning attempts—didn't look all that distasteful that day. I felt exposed as I became aware of our wealth. I regretted my past ungrateful thoughts about living with less than others.

The children's room with its wall-to-wall bunks revealed our easy western-style accumulation of things. Trinkets and toys found in the ship boutique, Christmas and birthday gifts lined the short shelves above their beds. Books, stuffed toys, china dolls, posters, Lego™, model cars, sports equipment and all the paraphernalia that exist in children's bedrooms back home suddenly seemed excessive as seen through their eyes.

Why did I feel strangely uncomfortable with showing them our lifestyle? Somewhere deep inside I was grappling with the unfairness of it all. I lived with plenty; they lived with scarcity. To our African friends we lived in a palace, yet when we showed our cabin to European friends, I felt their shock at our truly humble abode. To them we lived in an unbelievably tiny cabin and possessed almost nothing. I felt the stark contrast.

It wasn't until I visited Samba's home that I better understood the wonder filling his young wife's eyes as she toured our palace cabin. As I suspected, indeed, we were rich by comparison. Our arrival at their compound brought 30 smiling Africans to greet us. After this grand welcome, they eagerly escorted us to their simple dwelling. A tattered dirty curtain separated the bedroom from the main room of bare, chipped cement walls and floors. No doors to paint or hinges to oil in this home. No pictures on the walls or bookshelves to dust. No carpet to vacuum! An old clock solely furnished the room.

As they ushered our family in, Samba issued orders to retrieve cushions for the wooden frame of their couch. A parade of obedient children appeared from somewhere next door in the compound and slapped down the dusty inserts. I presumed that they'd been used as someone's mattress. These people's only assets appeared to be the many children running around the dusty compound.

One by one, members of Samba's family came inside to greet us, giving hearty welcomes and wide toothy grins. Although he had only three children, altogether he provided for six. Unemployed brothers dropped off nephews and nieces and he willingly cared for them. Aging parents, grandparents and aunts all lived together in one compound of which Samba seemed to be the head. This is the African way. Families provide for one another, care for one another and are linked inseparably for life. I remembered the verse from scripture: "God sets the lonely in families." This is the beauty and richness of a culture unlike our own; it is one of the blessings of being born African.

Obviously thrilled to have Westerners as guests, Samba spent what little money he had to serve us groundnuts, cashews and bottles of soda pop. We knew it stretched them to pay three Gambian Dalasi per bottle (about 35 cents). Samba set the refreshments on a wooden chair exclusively for his guests. Something felt dreadfully wrong with this scene. While we munched reluctantly on our delicious snacks, thirty Africans around us had nothing! The younger African children who didn't understand the occasion stared longingly at our treats. When Bruce offered nuts to the little ones, they reached, but their father shooed and reprimanded them. How heartbreaking and humbling to know that these children may never receive these simple luxuries, while ours could afford several soda pops each day!

Later they treated us to bananas and oranges from their yard. Never had we been given such hospitality and generosity at so great a cost to the host. With graciousness, we attempted to show our gratitude by accepting these gifts. Although we'd not been the surgeon who skilfully wielded the knife, we realized their gifts demonstrated their thankfulness for the kindness shown to their son by Mercy Ships. Mafugi's cleft lip no longer showed any signs of deformity since his surgery. Therefore, no longer was he doomed to life as a recluse without hope. Mafugi now had a future with opportunities and dreams like the other children. We shared their joy but felt humbled to receive such an offering of generosity extracted from poverty.

To amuse us, a young lad climbed the curved trunk of a coconut tree in their yard, and challenged Brandon to do the same. The African boy's lanky brown limbs wrapped easily and quickly around the trunk. Brandon followed his technique with a tad less skill and agility, but he couldn't reach the coconuts. A stronger teenage boy climbed stealthily towards the prize. We quickly cleared out of the way when it began to rain down coconuts. This kind of adventure seemed a far cry from skate-

Chapter Twenty Three

boards and roller blades, but Brandon enjoyed it just the same.

Samba led us to his deep well dug long ago in the middle of the compound. A rope and pail device supplied the lifeline for obtaining this precious commodity. During the dry season, neighbours also shared the well. Off to one corner of the compound, he proudly pointed out the luxury of cement showers where dirty privacy curtains hung sloppily. But the luxury came not from a showerhead, as we would suppose, but from a bucket. It appeared to be the only method of showering that they knew.

I spotted a run-down wooden shack in the corner of the compound, which slightly resembled a North American outhouse. When I questioned about its purpose, I felt shocked. Sadly, it turned out to be more living quarters for his family. The actual latrine looked even less appealing.

It triggered memories of my first repulsive experience with an African latrine. I had just begun a week of sterilizing instruments for the dental team. Although warned by the team leader about the unpleasantness of the local latrine, I put on my brave missionary resolve and set out down the road with the key. Unlocking the door, the rankness clutched my nostrils and took my breath away. Giant cockroaches with long, eerily twitching antenna seemed to size me up, then scurry and disappear to the dark corners. Looking up, I shuddered to see a spider the size of a man's hand on the ceiling. With my heart pounding and my body trembling with repulsion, I promptly closed the door and chose to find a less private, but less offensive alternative.

As we continued the tour of our host's peculiar yard, scrawny brown chickens strutted aside as we encroached on their territory. Even the chickens in Africa looked starved. As they pecked around the sandy floor of the walled compound, I inquired of

Samba as to what they were fed. "Would it be corn?" I asked trying to sound like a knowledgeable farm girl.

"Nothing," was the reply. "They feed themselves."

"Really?" I couldn't hide my surprise.

"They peck for food in the dirt," he answered. This struck me odd. As far as I could see, not one grain existed in that dirt. The naked ground would provide no meal for a chicken. Could there be microscopic bugs in this sand? I chose not to ask further. How could someone own livestock and not feed them? Then I remembered that people in this country had children they couldn't feed. Little wonder these chickens looked small and unhealthy compared to the fat free-range chickens I had seen butchered on my uncle's farm as a young girl. Yet another picture of the poverty of Africa. Existing within a walled compound of dry earth producing little food, like the chickens, the people daily pecked out a meagre survival.

Mealtime proved to be the greatest stretch for us in this cultural exchange. Samba, having seen the use of silverware on the ship, rounded up three tarnished mismatched spoons for us. Omit the use of napkins, placemats, or dinnerware of any kind. In fact, simply omit the use of a table altogether. At two in the afternoon, this family squatted around a gigantic dull, metal bowl for their mid-day meal. The bowl consisted of rice topped with something that resembled our galley scraps of fish. Steeling our stomachs we agreed to one taste since we'd already had our lunch on the ship. They laughed with great amusement as the "toubobs" (white folk) stooped to spoon some of their food. Obviously they understood this to be highly unusual for us.

So what do people use who cannot afford cutlery? Why, hands of course! Eagerly they all dipped into the community bowl.

Chapter Twenty Three

Somehow I had not recalled hearing any mothers calling kids to wash their hands before this meal. I could only trust God to protect us from any unfamiliar microscopic creatures entering our delicate systems in these unhygienic conditions.

Experiences such as this visit among the African people confirmed what I had heard and suspected. The strength of Africa is its people! Living in large extended families, tribal communities and villages, they shared their pain and sorrows, disease and hunger. They shared their triumphs, joys, and life's milestones. Not separated by large luxurious homes as in the western world, where neighbours are rarely seen or spoken to, loneliness seems less prominent in this part of the world. Burdens borne together somehow seem lighter. I had come to experience this truth in our Mercy Ship community.

We returned to our palace cabin on the ship that day. In tears, Bruce stopped to thank God for all that we had by contrast and for the opulence in which we lived. Our visit with these African friends shook off residual attitudes of self pity and discontentment with our simple lifestyle. The poor had humbled us.

A week later, Samba's four well-behaved children joined us at a table in the Mercy Ship dining room. In African cultures, children are taught to mind their manners and obey adults if they wished to avoid a beating. Samba gave clear instructions in their language on how to use a fork to eat their food from a plate. They appeared shy and awkward. We tried to reassure them with our smiles.

Eating slowly, they couldn't quite manage to finish the generous helping of strange Western institutional food placed before them. Taking their plates, Samba began to eat their leftovers. I assured him that he did not have to finish the remainder on their plates. I felt fairly certain that he had probably disliked our Western food.

"Food is food," he replied emphatically. I knew immediately that he would be offended by any waste. With that I began scraping together all the leftovers for him to take home in a plastic container. He was grateful. And he was right. Food is, indeed, food.

Cries of the Orphans

For crewmembers like us who worked on the ship, Mercy Ministries provided opportunities for service among the African people on the weekends. Our cell group chose to visit Mother Teresa's Sisters of Charity Home for malnourished babies. The newly-built sprawling complex appeared better equipped than any previous orphanages we'd seen in West Africa.

The faint odour of urine hung in the humid air as we entered a large room filled with steel cribs. One by one, tiny dark bodies lying on burgundy vinyl mattresses stirred, whimpered and cried for love and attention. We'd arrived after the morning nap when the routine of lifting weak, thin babies onto potties began. Most of the babies under the age of two wore terry cloth underwear. Often they'd soiled or wet the bare vinyl mattresses. Diapers are rarities in Africa.

Precious, sleepy babies sat hunched over on plastic potties— pink for the girls and green for the boys. Some cried at this heartless routine of being lifted by one arm and plunked down. Time did not permit cuddling or comforting. In fact, if the crying grew too loud, the African woman barked gruffly for them to stop. In fear, these babies sucked back the tears. How young they learn not to cry!

The next incident served to confirm an interesting fact shared in our medical receptions in Europe and South Africa. Generally people raised in a western nation without any formal medical training possess a higher knowledge of basic health care than those born in underdeveloped countries. For example, our mothers taught us to cleanse a cut or wound, and then bandage it. In parts of Africa, animal dung may be applied to the open cut or sore, unwittingly introducing further bacteria to the site.

At the orphanage, several babies suffered from an oozing yellow eye infection. While they squatted on their potties, the African woman used a wet wash cloth and proceeded to wipe every baby's eyes, without rinsing or changing cloths. The dear lady had no understanding that she actually spread the infection from baby to baby in this procedure.

Horrified, our Norwegian friend, Anne, tried to stop her and gently explained the ramifications of what she was doing. The language barrier made it difficult, and although the woman indicated that she understood, we suspected her set procedure would be no different the next day.

For this reason alone, I regarded our Community Health Teaching teams as a highly valuable ministry. The teams trained African people in health care, who in turn taught whole villages the basics in personal hygiene, wound care, sanitary food preparation, and clean water procedures. A diploma marked their weeks of education and practical learning. Such training served to save whole villages from disease and death. Along with helping those already afflicted, these are the lasting imprints of change that Mercy Ships seeks to make.

Beyond basic needs for physical survival, I witnessed the deeper needs of the human soul. The best illustration of this occurred when Bruce joined us at the orphanage. His presence created a fascinating scene. As soon as he sat on the floor, babies swarmed to him. They toddled, drooled, climbed and crawled over him. Drawn to him like bees to honey, he cuddled and wrestled with them. How the human heart cries for protection and provision, strength and security, love and affection from our fathers. As I watched this, I saw it as a clear expression of the heart's cry for daddy, Abba Father! Inwardly I thanked God for the gift of a caring, affectionate father for our children. Here in the orphanage, with both fathers and mothers absent, only basic physiological needs could be met by busy staff.

For several hours, our family held and played with precious malnourished babies desperately needing touch and attention. None of the staff had time for the luxury of affection, nor would they know the need of it for the babies' development.

Hearing their cries echo in our ears as we departed, we often drove home reflecting with sadness. Naturally we wondered if our weekly visits over those months would make a difference in their young lives. Liedeke, a child psychologist from Holland, assured us that it definitely would. Our attentions played a significant part in the steps towards healthy growth for many babies. Holding and affection, along with interactive play, fed and imparted the love and joy of Jesus to young hungry spirits. It had not been a difficult task.

Nevertheless, I always returned from those visits with a deep ache inside. My eyes took in the usual scenes on our route back to the ship—the dilapidated tin shacks, faded rags strewn over roofs to dry, goats and chickens wandering the red earthen roads, but my thoughts were gripped by orphans. Many, many, many are the orphans of Africa! Like locusts stealing and devouring the land, AIDS now rampantly kills the fathers and mothers of Africa.

Chapter Twenty Three

Precious young souls are left behind, alone in the world. Children just like these, crying for love.

The Father heart of God expresses love and compassion for widows and orphans. A new desire burned within me. We needed more people, more workers, more Christians willing to be the hands of the Father to care for the cries of the orphans. If only MORE people would sacrifice a LITTLE, it could make a BIG difference in this world. One life at a time.

Orphans impacted me like no others. These needy infants taught me to be humbly grateful for all that we have. Our blessings of home, education and prosperity were never to be taken lightly. With all these blessings, can we do anything less than simply love and care for the orphans?

24

Humbled by the poor

> *The brother in humble circumstances ought to take pride in his high position, and the one who is rich should take pride in his low position, because he will pass away like a wild flower.*
>
> James 1:9, 10

Since we longed for our families back home, our first Christmas living onboard heightened our homesickness. As the years passed, we grew to love and anticipate the wonderful traditions of the ship: the international Christmas Carol festival, open house cabins, a door decoration contest, cookie baking, Christmas worship services and the Dutch custom of filling shoes with gifts outside the door on Christmas Eve. The community of Mercy Ships became our loving family with whom we shared celebrations of the birth of our King.

Christmas gifts for our children and friends onboard had been purchased during the summer months while the ship was in Europe. The trick was to recall in which hold of the ship we'd stored them. One year we nearly gave up in despair, unable to find them. After that I learned to secretly record their location.

Little heads could be seen peeking out the cabin doors on Christmas morning. Peering down the long passageway of family cabins on Upper Deck, a heap of gifts lay stockpiled at each door. A thrilling time of giving onboard transpired late on Christmas Eve when crewmembers quietly stole about the ship dropping their gifts and cards into shoes. Small, meaningful gifts reflected the spirit of giving in a much deeper way than what we practised in our homelands.

While docked in Benin during our final Christmas onboard, we received a card with a mysterious anonymous note inside.

> Clue: Two legs good, four legs bad.
> Kids must find it in the port secured area.
> Mom can decide what to do with it and Dad can deal with it.

In response to Bruce's joking about chickens one day, fellow Canadian crewmember, Dave, conspired to enjoy the joke on him. Tied to a container in the port, the kids discovered a live russet-coloured chicken strutting about. Jillian named her *Henrietta* and took our unique Christmas gift for daily walks.

Pets are not allowed onboard, so after a week of feeding her galley corn on the dock, the family agreed to give her up to a needy home. Through our enquiries, we learned about Josephine.

Josephine, a widow with seven children, lived in a pathetic hovel in the middle of the city. For 37 years she existed in this squalor, a home unsafe and unfit for animals. Being a Christian woman, the church provided for her. One older son attending university would eventually bring a good income for this family. Another son lay dying of tuberculosis in a hospital.

Chapter Twenty Four

Bruce and I ducked into her dark hovel to deliver our chicken, all the while fearing the hut would collapse on top of us. Josephine met us bare-chested and sweating profusely in the hot, dank hollow she called home. Putting on a T-shirt, she continually wiped her glistening forehead and chest as we communicated through the pastor's translation.

My heart wrenched at the sight of such a woman. She pointed out the remains of her pepper mill which once supported the family when her husband was alive. Unable to fix it, her means of survival only took up space and collected dust. Her life since knew nothing but hardship and struggle for survival. Why hadn't God heard the prayers of this suffering woman? Or had he?

Pastor Christophe explained later that the church was in the process of building her a home. However, like many half-built structures in Africa, money ran out and the work ceased. I assured him I would try to do something.

Presenting the opportunity to our cell group and some friends in Europe, we agreed to raise funds for the continuation of this home. The home still needed a roof, doors and a bamboo fence. Little by little, I presented money to the pastor requesting receipts in return. Trust is a considerably difficult issue among the poor, even Christians. Poverty sometimes creates desperation and temptation.

Our next contact with Josephine occurred in temporary surroundings less decrepit than those of our initial meeting. She had moved out of her hovel into a hospital where she cared for her adult son suffering from tuberculosis. In West African hospitals, families are responsible for their loved one's meals and personal care. When Sue and I visited her in the hospital, she remarked with great hope that her son was doing much better. I had never encountered the sight of a grown man so emaciated. With Pastor Christophe leading, we began a prayer time around his bed.

Later in conversation, Josephine admitted that following her son's recovery, she hoped never to return to her home. She had reached the limit in that appalling existence. She'd also been given hope for a better life. Before we left, the pastor handed her some money, which I assumed came from the church. I felt miserable for not having any money with me that day to give her.

Near the end of our stay in Benin, moving day for Josephine finally arrived. Arranging for two Land Rovers and a flat bed truck, our willing cell group became movers. Through a ship-wide e-mail, I'd sent out a request for any furniture to help Josephine. Crew members donated a fine couch and chair along with some well-used furniture in a dock storage shed. I hesitated to send these latter pieces. They probably belonged in the city dump rather than a new home.

Sue had never seen Josephine's home until moving day. She turned to me and with her lovely New Zealand accent exclaimed breathlessly, "I'm speechless. I'm appalled! I can't even go in there. That's not fit for an animal!" I wholeheartedly shared her sentiments.

After loading up her belongings on the flatbed, Sigve from Norway, with a twinkle in his eye, expressed what we all felt, "Well, it looks like a load we would drive to the dump or use for firewood back home." We laughed with the sadness of it all. Then I felt pleased for having included the old furniture from the dock shed since it looked far better than anything Josephine owned.

Her empty hovel allowed the rats and cockroaches to take up sole residency. In all our travels among the poor, Josephine's home

Chapter Twenty Four

seemed to be the poorest of the poor. Excited to see the new home in which we'd carefully invested, initially I responded inwardly, "That's it?" I had expected more. Set in a rural area, this bamboo home had cement floors and a tin roof. We moved her furniture into the four rooms as she directed.

As the sun began to set, we paused for a photo together in front of her new home. Josephine expressed that she'd prayed and dreamed all her life for a house such as this. Her beaming face revealed her gratitude. We encouraged her to begin gardening in the land around her home. Ending with prayer for blessings and peace, we left her and her children to enjoy their new dwelling place. God had answered the prayers of an old widow beginning with a four-dollar Christmas chicken.

The poor of West Africa changed us. People like Samba's family humbled us by their generosity. An old widow and tiny orphans taught us to cease complaining and be more grateful for our blessings. We also discovered new treasure in the appreciation of richness in culture. Most of all, we gained a heightened sense of the humble privilege to be serving as a clay vessel, pouring out God's blessing to the poor of Africa!

Being born in a wealthy country, I pondered what it must be like to be born into a lifestyle of destitute poverty. Does it affect people's character and spirit? How does one live each day with such dire need and constant lack? Does this position of powerlessness and deprivation also choke character and produce a defeating sense of inferiority? I realized that these very questions reflected my Western point of view. I could compare the poor within a rich culture like Canada. The poor of Africa are a majority in their land and have experienced or seen no other alternative. (In some areas, however, television may be changing that fact.) When the rich and poor live together, there is the difficulty of comparison. Scripture implores the one in humble circumstances to take pride in his *high* position and the one who is rich to take pride in his low position. This had been a difficult perspective for *us* to assume during our years of difficulty in Canada.

Instead, I observed in the African poor, a tremendous resilience of the human spirit, demonstrating strength of character. The fierce love for one's family impressed me greatly. When a westerner begins to succeed materially, he enlarges his own lifestyle, moving up the independent ladder of wealth. When an African individual succeeds, he shares his abundance with family and community, raising the standard of living for all of them.

As I pondered people like Josephine, I felt further humbled. She suffered and persevered in unthinkable circumstances for most of her life. Yet, because of her hope in Jesus, she kept her head held high and her heart bowed low. Without bitterness, she hoped and boldly trusted God for provision. In fact, while we said our good-byes, she asked for more—someone to finance the repair of her pepper mill. Only days away from the ship's departure, and with an estimated cost of $400, we had to refuse her. In her mind, we seemed an endless supply of riches and God's provision. If only we could have been!

Days later, we left the poor behind us and sailed northward. Once again, we would dock among the world's wealthiest people. I wondered whether our hearts could be fully prepared for the contrast.

> A father to the fatherless, a defender of widows is God in his holy dwelling.
> Psalm 68:5

25

Honoured by the Rich

*He who is kind to the poor lends to the Lord,
and he will reward him for what he has done.*
Proverbs 19:17

Teodoro's Trumpet

A majestic island rising out of the sea lay shrouded in a milky, morning mist. The sun shone hazily through, brushing the volcanic mountains with a rusty red hue. White Spanish-style dwellings and palm trees clung to the lower mountainsides of Tenerife like tiny white mushrooms. From the rails of Promenade Deck, I immersed myself in this spectacular view beyond the sparkling Atlantic waters. As I breathed in deeply, fresh island breezes filled my lungs. The Mercy Ship sailed smoothly and noiselessly into the shores of Tenerife, Canary Islands. We prepared to dock for our familiar rest and refuel before heading north.

Once again I strained to hear the familiar sound of Teodoro's trumpet wafting over the waves. Each time we arrived we scanned the dock to find his lone, small figure. Tunes like *Amazing Grace* and *When the Saints Go Marching In* warmed our hearts and comforted our weary spirits. Over the years, Teodoro had become a precious friend dearly loved by the crew. Dedicated to welcoming and saluting the crew, he blessed us with his trumpet tunes both as we arrived and as we departed.

The Canary Islands, our haven of rest between sails to the "haves and have nots", provided a few days of relaxation for most crew. No inconvenient tour ropes blocked us; no supplies needed loading; no beggars tugged us at this gangway; no busy hospital or ministry schedules existed. The refuelling of the ship and replenishing of the crew began.

These retreat days offered time spent in the scriptures with passionate speakers to prepare us for the exciting yet daunting mission that lay ahead. Together, we became refreshed, renewed and united as one. The beauty of the island was also ours to explore. One side of the island offered lush green tropical views while the other presented volcanic landscapes and black beaches.

Our friend Teodoro found ways to bless the crew each time we arrived between the contrasting phases of our work. Free entrance to Loro Park, a fascinating zoo with vibrantly coloured parrots delighted and entertained us all. On another visit, Teodoro reserved a tour bus to drive us to the base of a volcanic mountain, the highest peak of the Spanish islands. As the owner and manager of a pizza business, one year he baked free pizza for the crew.

Chapter Twenty Five

Teodoro, a small-statured Salvation Army man living on a grand tourist island had become a great joy to hundreds of weary missionaries over the years. One year Teodoro and his trumpet didn't show up. Highly unusual, we knew something was amiss by his absence on the dock. Later, we learned that his dear wife lay dying of cancer. He apologized for overlooking our arrival. Crew responded to his grief by raising money to help with medical bills. This expression of love moved him to tears. One small man, one lone Christian, had regularly honoured an entire crew of missionaries by his resourceful generosity, his sweet, humble spirit and his musical gift. At last we could bless him in return.

A Hero's Welcome

The crew-missionaries appeared haggard, thin and weary. We had fought a five-month battle against heat and malaria, and against the enemy of God in a land of prominent Voodooism. The first Benin outreach had been far from smooth. Each step of the way wrought insufferable blows. Admittedly we were battle wounded and weary. It had been difficult for Mercy Ships to get into the country and then difficult to leave it.

To add to the matter, on the voyage back to Europe our usual period of rest in Tenerife turned into hard labour. Port authorities of Tenerife inspected our ship and demanded that the bilges (located below the engine rooms) be cleaned before passing us for departure. Crew volunteered by spending hours and days labouring in the engine room, instead of resting. I signed up for gangway watch, while Brandon donned three layers of clothing to reach into the smaller places of the oily bilges. He worked hard alongside adult crewmembers and returned soaked in oil from head to foot. Even his underwear had to be thrown away.

Sailing into the northern climate brought us to springtime in the United Kingdom. While the Welsh donned lighter apparel, most crewmembers wandered the decks shivering in their winter jackets. From sweltering Benin, where we'd experienced a weighty dose of harsh conditions, theft, greed, and corruption, we sailed into the port of Barry, Wales. Being our family's first return from an African country, we felt shocked by the grand place of honour and respect given us. Like soldiers welcomed home from war, we felt like heroes. Marching bands hailed us on the dock. The press esteemed our visit with favourable coverage. Churches welcomed us and offered warm-hearted hospitality.

A pastor and his wife became instant friends for our family. We savoured great food and relaxing fellowship in their home. Home cooked meals and fresh salads had long been forgotten in the daily ship fare of Africa. Further gestures of friendship and kindness in Wales amazed us. During the sail I had hoped to switch all our closets to warmer attire but due to a water shortage onboard, our laundry times had been cancelled. Heaps of musty clothing bulged from our closets. With all crewmembers facing this dilemma, it would mean weeks to catch up.

Geoff, a British officer who joined us temporarily in the deck department, felt so concerned about my backload of laundry that he insisted on taking it home in a green garbage bag. It returned to me washed and nicely folded. Along with it, he included a bucketful of new socks for Bruce. For our cabin, he donated a small table that belonged to his deceased grandfather. Generously he'd relinquished it to sail around the world with a missionary family.

On departure day from Wales, a care package arrived at the gangway for our family. It contained our favourite Welsh treats.

Our new friends sent it as a departing love gift. We valued these simple, homey gifts like great treasure, along with their friendship.

To end our visit, pastors around Barry rallied their church people to support and bid farewell to the Mercy Ship. A remarkably huge crowd of hundreds came to the dock to wave and cheer. They began to sing and shout songs of joy and hope as we departed. As we floated slowly down the river, the crowd that stretched along the dock ran beside us for a long period of time.

In our hearts, we saluted these wonderful followers of Christ in Wales who honoured us like heroes. Into our weary spirits, they'd poured their refreshing care. They likely had no idea what a healing balm they had been for us. We'd sailed into the port exhausted from giving; having received we left refreshed.

Hospitality of Holland

Summer weekends in foreign lands offered time to enjoy our host countries. Taking our family off the ship gave our children the freedom of lying in the grass, climbing trees and cycling narrow European streets. After five months in West Africa, where no parks exist, we took great delight in finding clean, wide open, grassy stretches. To add to the pleasure of our ship lunch in the park, we bought fresh apples and other fruits that we'd missed while in Africa.

For this mom, the time in Holland meant a shopping quest to prepare for the five months ahead. Filling our cupboards with inexpensive, healthy food snacks and finding gifts to stash away for birthdays and Christmas, demanded a lot of pavement time.

Nevertheless, when I think of the Netherlands, I remember the quaint countryside dotted with windmills, the meandering canals, dikes and bicycle pathways. But most of all, I remember the people with whom we connected so deeply. During the cultural orientation for crew upon arrival, we'd been informed that the Dutch people may seem resistant at first, but when their loyalty is won, a friend is gained for life. How true that turned out to be!

Four families from the province of Groningen, in the northern part of the Netherlands, hosted our family during our short visit. Each one blessed us with their friendship and generous hospitality. Before we left Holland, our new friends, Bert and Ria, arrived at the ship loaded with a cart full of practical supplies for Africa. They had collected gifts for the children, perfumes and soaps for Bruce and me. During one short visit, they presented a bicycle and roller blades. Beyond all this expression of love through gifts, we treasured their friendship most of all.

Our friendship with Bert triggered great changes in his life. Jolted out of complacency, God began to soften his heart. In the two years between our visits, we saw a remarkable change in his marriage, in his commitment and hunger for God. Today he serves God with joy and fervour.

Aside from pouring ourselves into the work of medical and press receptions, pastors and ladies' teas, youth events and tours for thousands, it was also individuals like Bert, changed by the ministry of Mercy Ships, that made the journey to Europe so exciting. The main purpose for our visit was to promote public awareness, procure supplies and recruit crew for Africa, but our lives also impacted others.

From port to port as the Mercy Ship docked its pristine, white hull, thousands came aboard to see the miracle hospital ship. While touring, they also heard about the greater miracle of Christ transforming lives. Some came to know the Saviour through these tours onboard. We met a Dutch man whose spiritual destiny had been changed forever by the visit of Mercy Ships four years earlier.

The hospitality of Holland through the warm-hearted people left a strong impression on our family. Our children realized that though we had sacrificed our family and friends back home to give to the poor, God abundantly poured out His love through others in return. We came into a port as strangers and left with many new friends.

The Nature of Norway

Breathtakingly beautiful fjords, waterfalls, grassy mountains and colourful historic street fronts shattered our icy images of Norway. We also discovered its people far from being icy and cold! Norwegians acquired the reputation for the most generous, charitable nation to Mercy Ships in Europe.

Our family felt grateful for all our experiences among the Norwegians. One typical hearty-looking Norseman from near Stavanger invited several crewmembers to his family cabin. A part of the journey took us across a lake in a rowboat to his rustic, charming cabin perched part way up the mountain. To meet warm, open people of another culture is a pleasure; to experience their hospitality is an even greater privilege.

Another generous host guided us on a bus tour up the fjords while the ship docked in the port town of Bergen. A misty day created endless scenes of picturesque waterfalls cascading down the cliffs. Playing softly in the background, symphony music of Norwegian classical composer, Edvard Greig, enhanced the beauty. Traversing the mountainous heights in the safety of the bus, we peered raptly below at the zigzagging roads we'd left behind. We left awe-struck by the wonders of God's diverse creation.

Aside from sightseeing and daily ministry onboard, there were numerous opportunities to share the work of Mercy Ships in the port communities. *"Declaring the marvellous deeds of God among the people,"* as the Psalmist proclaims, became for us an enjoyable part of the ministry. Brandon, age ten, answered questions in a Norwegian Sunday school with the help of a translator. Appointed as guest speakers, Bruce and I hosted an evening dinner presentation of Mercy Ships at a large church gathering. In appreciation, they presented me with a striking bouquet of bright yellow sunflowers. Strongly accented by my deep blue African suit, I felt drenched in God's outpouring love that night.

Being in a northern climate once again, Bruce's thoughts turned towards hockey. Spending the majority of the year in Africa did not lend itself to teaching certain types of sports in Physical Education class. Seizing the opportunity, he navigated his way around the daunting freeways and tunnels of Norway. He hoped to find an arena to secure some ice time for his students. To his great joy, the opportunity was granted completely free! With feverish excitement, many of his students stood on ice skates for the first time. For those few sessions, Bruce taught the rules of ice hockey and enjoyed several games. Along with the students, the teacher was in his glory! It seemed a special provision for a Canadian boy who'd missed the ice for three and a half years while in missions.

Norway's dramatic scenery and friendly people encouraged and inspired us all. Indeed in every country we discovered God's distinctive fingerprint of beauty and creativity, as well as His remnant of people who loved and served Him. Through these fellow believers, our family received care and refreshment; we valued home-cooked meals, gifts, trumpet salutes, personal retreats, hot baths, sightseeing and friendship.

Chapter Twenty Five

Blessed to Bless Others

As missionaries, we had learned about God's true economy of giving and receiving. Praying and trusting Him for both the big and little things became our common way of life. As we cheerfully gave to others, it seemed His abundance continually poured out to us. It is true that we are blessed to bless others.

Paula Kirby is a Trinidadian lady and former dancer whom I saw consistently live out this principle onboard. Encountering her standing at the gangway one day, I prattled admiringly over her African dress. She wore it elegantly and I naturally complimented her. Then, feeling impulsive, I teasingly quipped, "Isn't there some country or culture where you compliment a person on something and they have to give it to you?" After it rolled off my tongue, I felt embarrassed and wished my silly words could have been retrieved. We laughed.

The next day, a brown package appeared at my cabin door with the following note: *"There is such a country—it's called the kingdom of God. A place where we are blessed to bless others. Love Paula."* Instantly I recalled my impulsive words. Before I even opened the package, I knew what was inside—the beautiful African dress. Gratefulness welled up into tears. I was speechless for a long time.

I wore the dress often. Before leaving the ship, I lovingly passed it on to another gal. Not only had the dress spiced up my tired, outdated wardrobe, but it had served to remind me of the Kingdom of God—a place where we are blessed to bless others.

Churches caught this vision and renewed their passion for the poor and lost. Generosity abounded in the wealthy nations where we implored the rich to give to the poor. Deck hands painstakingly loaded donated construction materials and medical supplies deep into the holds of the hull. Crewmembers formed a human chain from the dock down to the stores, passing boxes of food. Soon the Mercy Ship was fully loaded in preparation for our return to the poorest of the poor in West Africa.

 Finally, we bade farewell to our last port of call, farewell to the peoples of Europe who generously gave of their time, their money and their resources. With each new port, we had encountered another language, another currency and another people. Our travels filled our treasury with new friends and experiences. Truly, we had been honoured by the rich and extravagantly blessed to see God's amazing world from the portholes of an older ship. A ship purposed to serve and bless others, in so many ways blessed us!

26

School of Mercy

The quality of mercy is not strained
It droppeth as the gentle rain from heaven
Upon the place beneath: it is twice blessed;
It blesses him that gives and him that takes…
    William Shakespeare – Merchant of Venice

Summoned from a small town in Ontario, then stationed aboard a ship, these clay vessels had much to learn about the true meaning of mercy. Far from being flawless clay vessels, the abiding, loving Potter's work persisted in our lives as we served. To truly understand mercy, God enrolled us in a school filled with practical experiences. In this gracious school of mercy, His lessons changed our lives.

MERCY 101: "Let Mercy Triumph Over Judgment"
- James 2:13

Lightly visible heat waves sizzled and rebounded off the concrete and earthen roads as Brandon and Bruce walked into the town of Cotonou, Benin. As they arrived at the market, their white skin attracted street sellers. Offering belts, wallets, CD's, toothbrushes, postcards and the like, suddenly the two found themselves surrounded by aggressive, young African men.

The crowd of bargainers grew more intense and the circle began to close in around the two. Being shorter, ten-year-old Brandon couldn't see overtop of the crowd. He tightened his grip on his dad's arm as he grew more nervous and fearful. Turning, they seized an opportunity to duck into the closest store. The sellers remained outside. Once Brandon caught his breath and calmed himself, they escaped. Unfortunately, this initial experience with the ways of African culture left Brandon frightened and leery of its people for much of our time in missions.

To the street seller in this French African culture, a "non merci" simply meant he needed to bargain harder and be more persuasive. Repeating "Non!" several times with no eye contact proved unsuccessful in fending them off. Walking quickly, as though deaf and mute seemed to help us escape the barrage. Sometimes we left a trail of disappointed vendors behind us.

Women in the markets grabbed my arm trying to persuade me to visit their booths. The touching, jostling, grabbing and begging rankled my nerves and pushed my senses into overload. By the end of my market walks, I felt annoyed and indignant with these people.

Why couldn't they respect my answer? Why did they have to

be so aggressive? Couldn't they see that their pushiness made me feel violated and angry? Where is their personal dignity that they need to approach me with offensive selling tactics? Their forceful ways grew increasingly repulsive to me.

A similar experience happened in Guinea. Being white and therefore considered rich, a taxi driver heavily overcharged me. My African translator attempted to correct this injustice by reasoning with the driver. A policeman stood on the corner overhearing the conversation. I felt mortified when a loud yelling match in French ensued over the issue. To my chagrin, the policeman sided with the taxi driver insisting that I pay. He gestured strongly towards my purse to which I responded reluctantly. The injustice bothered me, but I wasn't about to risk being thrown in jail over it.

To most Africans, this is perfectly just. Being white-skinned and therefore rich, I must pay more. As a missionary, living on a meagre income by my country's standards, this perturbed me.

On another occasion, I walked home from a market jaunt in The Gambia with my girlfriend and a few of our children. I had trained myself to always be aware of my small shoulder purse which bobbed at my side. Instantly I recognized the sound of the Velcro flap being opened. Heavy crowds were meant to disguise the pick-pocketer's attempt. I grabbed his arm directly, looked my thief in the face and yelled, "Don't you ever try that again!" My adrenaline surged and people stopped and stared as I lectured this young man towering above me. He shook my hand and apologized for his wrongdoing while slowly trying to dismiss himself.

As we walked back to the ship, we laughed away the tension. My reaction in the face of violation and personal injustice shocked me, as well as the children. Who was this gentle mother who growled like a bear when attacked! "Go Mom!" teased my boys. Having gained familiarity with African ways, Brandon walked a step behind me and kept a watchful eye like a queen's guard.

As my frustrations grew, so did my attitude of superiority and judgment. It seemed that at every turn we faced pathetic incompetence, unnecessary hassles, injustice, corruption and senseless ways of doing things. I discovered a saying that obviously transpired out of frustration from foreigner's inability to forge through the many hold-ups and setbacks in these countries. 'WAWA' stood for *West Africa Wins Again!* The picture is one of throwing hands up in resignation and shaking heads at the futility of it all.

In pouring out all these frustrations to the Lord, I felt ashamed admitting, "God, I'm not sure I love these people." *How could I reach a people whom I found offensive?*

Slowly God revealed to me that I would remain frustrated if I continued to view them through my Western eyes and mind set. I needed to take off my Canadian glasses and learn to adapt to a culture that thinks and acts differently from my own. Rather than getting caught up in judging what they did as right or wrong, I needed to be concerned with showing the mercy of God. Instead of wasting energy brooding about my personal offences, I needed to love as Christ loved.

I also felt convicted to stop using the 'WAWA' expression and trust God to work through every situation. My personal pride, rights and shameful attitude of superiority had to be laid down if I wanted to cross the bridge to this culture.

I expected to experience culture shock, but I had not counted on the Lord revealing my own pride and prejudices through it.

Chapter Twenty Six

My liberation came in asking Christ to love the African people through me. Asking for a spirit of mercy to triumph over judgment became my constant prayer. Only then did I experience an inner change that allowed my ministry among the people of Africa to bear fruit.

A Dutch receptionist crewmember sent this fitting and timely e-mail to the crew during that first outreach to Benin. I changed the nationality to reflect my own background and kept it to remind myself of the need for an attitude of humility.

I Corinthians 13 - *A Guide to Culture*

- If I speak with the tongue of a national, but have not love, I am only a resounding gong or a clanging cymbal.

- If I wear the national dress and understand the culture and all forms of etiquette, and if I copy all mannerisms so that I could pass for a national but have not love, I am nothing.

- If I give all I possess to the poor, and if I spend my energy without reserve, but have not love, I gain nothing.

- Love endures long hours of language study and is kind to those who mock his accent; love does not envy those who stayed home; love does not exalt his home culture, is not proud of his national superiority, does not boast about the way we do it back home, does not seek his own ways, is not easily provoked into telling about the beauty of his home country, does not think evil about this culture.

- Love bears all criticism about his home culture, believes all good things about this new culture, confidently anticipates being at home in this place, endures all inconveniences.

- Love never fails; but where there is cultural anthropology, it will fail; where there is contextualization it will lead to syncretism; where there is linguistics, it will change.

- For we know only part of the culture and we minister to only part, but when Christ is reproduced in this culture, then our inadequacies will be insignificant.

- When I was in Canada, I spoke as a Canadian person, I understood as a Canadian person, I thought as a Canadian person, but when I left Canada I put away my Canadian things.

- Now we adapt to this culture awkwardly; but He will live in it intimately; now I speak with a strange accent, but He will speak to the heart.

- And now these three remain, cultural adaptation, language study, and love, but the greatest of these is LOVE.

MERCY 102: "That's What Mercy Is - Undeserved"

Some of our early lessons in mercy seem simple from this vantage point, but in the midst of crises and struggles, the view appeared quite different.

Even for seasoned missionaries the first outreach to Benin proved to be an extreme challenge. In the broader picture, the struggles began before entering the nation. Advance team members met with opposition and difficulty at every turn. Benin's Christian president had invited us to come, but evidently the warm invitation didn't filter down through all levels of his government. Getting the protocol signed became laborious. Co-operation at other levels proved tedious and frustrating.

Voodoo priests, upon hearing of our arrival threatened to protest on the dock. Herein lay the picture of the true battle in the heavenlies. Satan vehemently opposed our presence in a country boasting the birthplace of Voodoo, a religion practiced to this day. His domain and territory came under siege by the arrival of Mercy Ships. The mercy of Christ pouring into villages would affect areas of Voodoo strongholds. Missionaries already labouring in Benin thanked us for our strong presence to boost their efforts. The arrival of 350 more missionaries accelerated their work tremendously.

Priests of the Voodoo religion possess demonic power strong enough to curse people with sickness or even death. Many Beninois Africans live in fear of vengeful gods. They build altars and booths to offer food, and pay priests to protect them.

Through the spiritualism of Africa, I gained an awareness of how little we as Christians in the Western world are discerning of the spirit world. Focusing mainly on the material world, we forget that as scripture states, our battle is not against flesh and blood but against principalities and powers in the unseen world (Eph. 6:10). Unblocked by scientifically trained minds, most Africans are fully aware of this realm. How ironic that we as Christians who've been enlightened and given the answer to the powers of darkness, live in unbelief and ignorance, while they, knowing its dark power, have no light.

Aside from the lack of port security upon arrival, we immediately encountered other obstacles. Demanding a bribe, Benin custom officers refused to release our ship cargo for weeks after arrival. Because of the policy of Mercy Ships not to deal in bribes, our construction teams got off to a late start. Consequently the building project remained unfinished at the end of our stay. One crewmember graciously stayed behind to complete it. Furthermore, dental teams worked valiantly despite being forced to do examinations without proper equipment, while it lay stored in the holds of the ship awaiting release from customs agents. A host of people missed opportunities for care because of the greed of a few top officials.

Portholes on the lowest deck and in the school area required a wire cover to prevent theft. Officers and night patrols spotted sly signals between thieves on the dock and warded off their attempts. Even attempts to climb up the mooring ropes could only be thwarted by deck hands using water hoses on the offenders. Despite our efforts, deep in the night, robbers noiselessly stole bikes off the racks on aft deck and tossed them overboard to the waiting boats below. Sometimes smaller boys in canoes alongside the ship squeezed through a porthole to snatch anything of value inside.

Berthed by an unsecured pier, it became difficult to guard our vehicles. Hiring a young African lad to both assist our mechanic and guard the vehicles worked favourably for a time. Then mysteriously, parts began to disappear off the vans and Land Rovers. Our large Ford Econoline van was likely the only one in the country. It would have taken months to ship parts from the USA. Undeterred, our clever, good-humoured American mechanic ventured to Cotonou's marketplace—the largest in West Africa. There he found the elusive Ford van parts and bought them back. Regularly he purchased the stolen parts in the market. Soon he discovered that our young guard had found himself a secondary job—selling parts from our vehicles to other Africans. He, who had become a trusted friend of the crew, was dismissed in love. Mercifully, we didn't hand him over to the authorities to be beaten or put in prison.

In addition to these troubles, crew mourned the loss of two patients who died in the ward that year—a highly unusual event for Mercy Ships. The unbearable heat on the ship, and the lack of promised port security made it an outreach rife with hardship and struggle.

Chapter Twenty Six

By the end of our time in Benin, most crewmembers counted down the days, hours and then minutes to our departure. Days before, trouble began to brew. A misunderstanding between our purser and port agent resulted in a huge setback. Hours prior to leaving, African friends gathered and crowded on the dock in the hot sun to bid us farewell. Dancers and musicians showed their appreciation through performances. The departure time of 1400 hours came and went while we leaned on the rails of Promenade Deck longing for cooler temperatures and wondering what went wrong.

An announcement gave sketchy details about a problem with tugboats. Three hours later, the enthusiastic crowds on the dock dwindled. Our CEO, Simonne Dyer, taxied into town to negotiate with the customs officers and port agent who had refused to send tugs. Although our protocol states that we are exempt from departure taxes, we'd been slapped with a US $12,000 tax. With absolute firmness, Simonne refused to pay and said she would take this to the Office of the President. Finally she returned to the waiting crew and gave the victory signal on the dock.

As I sat at a table on deck, I found myself again questioning the attitudes and corruption of these people. How could they even think of asking for more money? Instead of thanks, they continued to strip us of all our resources. Our sacrificial crew, a "walking fresh blood bank" for the patients, had sweated profusely and shed many a tear. Quite literally, our blood, sweat and tears flowed in Benin. I seethed at the rudeness and ingratitude!

Crossing my arms, I arrived at this firm conclusion: "This country did not even deserve the Mercy Ship coming to help." At this point the Holy Spirit spoke clearly. *That's what mercy is. Undeserved. You are* **Mercy** *Ships.*

The revelation went further. Mercy is not at all dependent on the attitude of the recipient. In fact, an erring recipient comes into greater need of mercy by his or her misdeeds. It is not dependent on the response of the one receiving it. Mercy prevails whether we have our faces rudely spat in, or are shown appreciation. The reason for offering mercy lies in the fact of the need and in the mandate of Jesus to be merciful.

We are all undeserving of mercy. From a universal viewpoint, God has chosen not to give us what we deserve—hell. Instead He offers to give us what we don't deserve—heaven. Herein stands the greatest mercy of all! His free gift of salvation. In place of death and hell, mercy sent Jesus to a hideous cross for us. That we continue to walk and breathe daily is only a direct result of His mercy.

His mercy still flows unceasingly. Like the sea, it flows over our lives wave upon wave upon wave. Steady, rhythmical and ever present in our world today is the mercy of our great God. Like the enduring oceans, its endless flow often goes unnoticed. However, we would be doomed if the waves of mercy ever ceased.

Five hours after our scheduled departure time, we finally sailed away from Benin. Refreshing cooler offshore breezes greeted and soothed the deflated crew. Peering back at Benin, I left behind the anger and bitterness towards its people. Mercy had flooded my heart and washed it away.

27

Mercy Hands

She opens her arms to the poor and extends her hands to the needy.

Proverbs 31:20

MERCY 201: Mercy Hands Open Doors

According to Fredrick Faber, "Kindness has converted more sinners than zeal, eloquence, and learning." In the small country of The Gambia, we saw this concept in action. As Mercy Ministry teams dispatched their crew into the country week after week in small acts of kindness, changes occurred in this Muslim nation.

Beaches in the Republic of The Gambia are a huge resource

for tourism. Many of the Gambian people are sustained totally by the tourism industry. Garbage and litter turn these lovely beaches into unsightly, uninviting spots. Seeing the need, crewmembers spent hours picking up the garbage on beaches and stadium grounds. Unheard of in a land where white European visitors are to be served in hotels and luxurious resorts, the people's hearts stirred. This simple act of kindness drew photographers and journalists who wrote favourable articles about the Christians of Mercy Ships. The people raised us to a place of respect and honour.

A Gambian man commented, "That ship is good. Even though I am a Muslim, I can see the good things that have come from there. The locals here are very superstitious. In the evenings, they come out to stare at the ship. They say they can see angels covering her."

Initially our crewmember teams were forbidden to enter a Gambian prison with puppets and music. Seeing the depressing conditions of the prisons, Steve, the team coordinator, instead asked permission to have the teams paint the walls. With this new offer, officials granted permission. While painting week after week, crew members interacted and reached out to destitute prisoners. Even the guard's affection for our team grew.

Once favour had been won by a simple act of mercy, the director of the prison invited the teams to come. Puppets, drama and music teams entered the forbidden prisons to present the Christian message. One by one, Jesus moved among the captives and set them free. Weekly Bible studies and singing brought joy to sad, hopeless countenances. The transformation on the newly painted walls reflected in the hearts of the occupants. Prisoners longing for freedom *from* those walls, found freedom *within* the walls.

The head warden lifted a strict ban on Christians visiting prisons in all of The Gambia! Churches and missionaries are now free to enter and proclaim Christ in the local prisons. Pastors' wives presently visit the women's division of prisons. This experience impressed me as strong proof that "mercy hands" open doors to minister the gospel, even prison doors!

Access to medical care, surgery, and dentistry is unavailable for most of the poor of West Africa. The need for our services is far greater than we could ever meet! Therefore, invitations to West African countries are long-standing. Muslim countries, otherwise reluctant to allow Christians, open their doors to Mercy Ships due to their great need of the services offered. Further evidence that the hand of mercy can open many doors; these doors provide opportunities to speak into the eternal needs of people.

At times, responding to the vast need for acts of mercy felt like only a drop in the ocean. God's waves of mercy flowed over the sea of humanity as we administered hope and healing one life at a time.

MERCY 202: Show and Tell Gospel

Without the message of Christ prompting inward personal transformation and altering worldviews, change is difficult in places like Africa. The curse of poverty sometimes lies in the spiritual strongholds of animism, voodoo, and idolatry. Fatalistic beliefs and cyclical thinking that offer no future or hope keep many of the poor bound in their ways. Without a vision or hope, the people perish, as stated in Proverbs 29:18.

Don Stephens, founder of Mercy Ships describes this phenomenon in his book *Mandate for Mercy*.

John Mbiti, a philosopher and theologian from Kenya, has done extensive research on 270 different language groups in Africa (not dialects, but entirely separate language groups). In all 270 language groups, he has not found a single word for "future." Each of those language groups reflects a culture that does not see the events of life as moving forward, but rather as moving in cycles. There are the cycles of the rainy season and the dry season, birth and death, planting and reaping. Since everything moves in cycles, there is no real future, just cyclical toil. So there is no real need to convey such a concept as "future." And the absence ties the people to their cyclic, fatalistic, world view.

How different is the Christian world view! For Christians, history is going somewhere. We draw from the past, build in the present, and plan for the future.

The essence of the gospel is that we have a beginning, we were created, and the decisions we make during our life will affect our future. The gospel also speaks of God redeeming our past, becoming an active partner with us in this life, and securing for us a future hope.

It is simple and wonderful. It is what marks Christianity as unique from all other world views. And one of the most effective ways I know to bring people face to face with the truth of the gospel and the Christian world view is through simple acts of mercy and kindness.[1]

In a world full of many wonderful humanitarian and Christian organizations, I am perplexed over the reality that the problems of Africa have not been solved through the years. Many secularists believe education to be the key to making lasting change. I agree that this is one of the components. However, lasting transformation only begins when God redeems a culture through His work of grace. As belief systems change through the renewing of the mind, people begin to work towards a hope and a future for this life and for the next.

Chapter Twenty Seven

For this reason, evangelists and teachers travelled alongside medical, dental, construction, and water and sanitation teams. *The Decayed Tooth, Decayed Heart* story of the dental team clearly combined the message for body and spirit. People quickly understood the pain of a rotten tooth paralleled with the decay of sin in our lives. The story proved highly compelling and powerful. Numerous people asked for prayer or came to put their faith in Christ.

Many Christians and organizations tend to use only one means of expressing the gospel. Showing acts of mercy is easier for some Christians, causing them to overlook the need for proclamation of the gospel. This is like offering a cup of cold water, but not telling whose name it is in. Leaving Jesus out of the equation is to become wonderfully humanitarian, changing lives only on this side of eternity.

On the other hand, evangelism through the telling of the gospel is far less effective without the modelling of mercy. A "faith without works" is a dead faith, James warns in his epistle (James 2:17). Hand in hand, word and deed work successfully, caring for both body and spirit. Jesus, himself both healed and taught. His acts of mercy demonstrated the Fatherheart of God while His teaching offered restored relationship with God. By expressing the gospel message through showing and telling, change occurs for this life and for eternity.

Week by week on the floating hospital, department heads of medical, dental, health education, community development and evangelism reported the heart and hands of the ministry—both triumphs and tragedies—with all crewmembers. Not once did I sit through a session without fighting back the tears. The success of God working through these clay vessels using the two-handed expression of the gospel message, both show and tell, was always utterly amazing and miraculous!

Our lessons in the school of mercy not only challenged but inspired us. Yet it was only the beginning of learning to apply them to our lives.

28

Mercy for Missionaries

He has showed you, O man, what is good. And what does the Lord require of you? To act justly and to love mercy and to walk humbly with your God.

Micah 6:8

MERCY 301: The Harvest of Mercy

Breaking the chains of darkness in places like Africa requires spiritual perseverance and toil. Intercessory prayer and worship prepares the way for Christian workers and missionaries. Our first entry to Benin seemed to demonstrate our lack of preparation in the spiritual realm. We'd been unprepared for the severe nature of the battle.

Although we felt defeated, we later understood that the unseen realm may have shown a different perspective. An educated

Beninois man visiting in England met one of our medical staff and remarked enthusiastically, "Ah, you are from the Mercy Ship? There has been a big change in our country since you visited! You can even feel the difference." *Could this be true?* We doubted.

Three years later, when leaders announced our return to Benin, a heavy sigh released quietly from the crew. Memories of the struggle had not been forgotten. "Why was God asking us to revisit Benin, of all places?" many voiced openly. The President of Benin pleaded for our return and this time assured us of his promises for ease and security. For our family, the outreach would be our last before leaving the Mercy Ship to return to Canada.

Earnest prayer began after the announcement of our return. Early bird prayer warriors rose to the challenge. Then, on November 04, 2000, worship dancers and banners on aft deck unfurled and flowed while the Mercy Ship drifted into the port of Cotonou for the second time. Knowing what to expect gave the crew an edge. This time we felt far better equipped for the battle. Much prayer and worship, surrender and zeal abounded and surged towards this country.

Even the landscape seemed different upon arrival. Our visual memories of Benin rendered images of drought—dusty reddish brown earth with thirsty trees and no grass. Not so this time! Flourishing palm trees and green grass covered boulevards lining the streets. Evidence of maintenance and care in the city astonished us. A newly paved highway replaced a rutted, rambling road. Intense bottlenecks of traffic flowed more freely. Although still ravaged by poverty, the country's industry and commerce had grown. It all looked cleaner, greener and somehow more hopeful. We also learned of a struggling 40-member church now exploding at 400! God clearly worked in this nation and it was changing!

Chapter Twenty Eight

Surprisingly, a prime berth awaited us, designated for the Mercy Ship. Securing the port area with containers, armed security guarded us around the clock. Faithfully, these men kept us protected for the entire seven months, surpassing all efforts in previous ports. A large sign with bold letters outside the port read:

> By invitation of the President of Benin, the hospital ship M/V Anastasis, Mercy Ships.

In contrast to our previous visit, we felt acknowledged, welcomed and treated with special care. Even though the country faced severe fuel shortages, the president arranged for a diesel tank to be delivered to our ship port area. This enabled our ministry teams to fill their vehicles and do their work unhindered. It proved to be a tremendous blessing to us and thus to the poor.

Just as Elisha prayed for his servant's eyes to be opened to the host of horses and chariots surrounding them, we too longed to see this land through spiritual eyes. It seemed that the territory for our work had been enlarged and the fields ploughed by our first visit. Was it any wonder that it proved so hard and laborious? With the land subdued, seeds planted lay ready for watering and tending. This time the crew of Mercy Ships reaped a glorious harvest for the kingdom of God in Benin.

Sometimes God asks us to revisit the hard places in our lives. Only then can He bring healing and blessing. By resisting, we can actually miss out on His blessings and plans for us. Our return showed us the powerful hand of God at work in unseen ways. Our first visit had not been in vain. Concurring with former CEO Simonne Dyer, I believe that suffering and sacrifice eventually releases blessing. The toilsome, painful work of showing mercy eventually reaped a harvest for the Kingdom in Benin.

MERCY 302: Mercy for Meyers

Like flowers in a greenhouse, the protection and warmth of community life allowed people to flourish and grow in unprecedented ways. While I chafed at the immaturity allowed in our ranks of service, I soon came to see this as the great blessing of mercy.

Mercy Ships is open and accepting of many levels of spiritual and emotional maturity among those serving as crewmembers. Occasionally that created needless conflict, but mostly it proved to be a valuable time of growth and discipleship. If our God is even more merciful than this, who am I to judge whom He chooses to send? Only by the refining fires of His love and because of His great mercy did we ourselves share the privilege to be onboard.

Following one stressful time of work, my body crashed in fatigue requiring several days off work. Returning, I admitted my feelings to my boss, a young American woman, "I feel so guilty about being ill here onboard."

"What on earth for?" Kendra responded.

"Because my thyroid condition is a weakness. When I'm not careful enough, I'm no longer an asset to the ministry of Mercy Ships."

"But we all have areas in our lives that are not up to par, whether it be a physical weakness, emotional setbacks, troubles and burdens of home, homesickness or areas of sin. Few of us are completely strong people, but God uses us despite our areas of weakness. Yours just happens to be your health. But that doesn't mean you aren't an asset to the ministry or useful to God," she explained reassuringly.

Her insightful, wise response remained with me as evidence of God's mercy for all missionaries. It washed over my guilt like

Chapter Twenty Eight

healing waves.

Despite Bruce's Hepatitis C, he remained in good health throughout our time in missions. We soon discovered why just months prior to returning to Canada!

Knowing of Bruce's disease, one day the lab technician approached him. "I've just received a new test for Hepatitis C onboard. Can I test it out on you?" Colleen asked lightly. Bruce quickly agreed.

The results bewildered us. The test returned negative, causing the lab technician to doubt the new test's effectiveness. But it raised new hope in our minds. Could it be possible that Bruce had been miraculously healed? Doubts kept us in suspense when a second test arose as the result of a recurrent difficult incident in our lives.

Two months prior to leaving the Mercy Ship for home, a student approached me in the dining room as I carried my lunch tray and asked, "Did you know they are carrying Bruce up the gangway?"

"Oh no, not again!" I responded. Somehow I knew instantly that his knee had been re-injured. This time he had been teaching a Physical Education class European handball off ship. The memories of the last ordeal with knee surgery quickly surfaced.

For the third time, the same knee required surgery. The ship's medical insurance company booked our flights and arranged for surgery in London, England. Hastily, we made arrangements for the care of our children. Days later, I flew with Bruce from Benin to London, England. An extensive ACL knee operation was scheduled days after arrival. On the desk of our new British surgeon sat the results of blood tests taken a day earlier. While the surgeon got called out of the office briefly, Bruce leaned over to see the results for the Hepatitis C test.

Negative! Mysterious and miraculous! We stared at each other in amazement.

Three subsequent blood tests have since returned negative, puzzling doctors in Canada. Specialists explained to Bruce that the disease can go into remission but the results always remain positive on blood tests. His results are unexplainably negative.

Exactly when it happened, we are not certain. Some time during our missionary service, Bruce became the recipient of a miracle of God. We had sacrificed to serve on a *Mercy Ship of hope and healing* and in the process had received both ourselves!

Did we ever graduate from the school of mercy? For me, it appears to be a school of a lifetime. I am more naturally bent to see the wrongdoing, ascribe blame and then judge. But my desire is to season justice with mercy.

The supreme lesson in mercy came through receiving it ourselves. It fell quietly and gently. So quietly, we almost missed it, had it not been for that mishap near the end of our service.

29

Remember the poor

> *"For I was hungry and you gave me something to drink, I was a stranger and you invited me in, I needed clothes and you clothed me, I was in prison and you came to visit me."*
>
> Matthew 25: 35, 36

A gnawing guilt grew inside me as our departure date drew nearer. Our family would be leaving Mercy Ships after four years of ministry to the poor. God had fulfilled His purposes through us and we knew it was His timing for our family to return to Canada. Yet, how could we return to our wealthy country while Africa still remained poor and needy?

Positioning myself strategically for a view from the pool deck, I spent time wrestling with these issues as I met with God. While watching the activity below, my heart began to break. On the starboard side of our ship, below the hazy equatorial sun, men in crude fishing boats paddled out to the ocean. On the port side, shirtless, sweating African men dressed in frayed pants scrambled around the dock unloading rice from a huge bulk carrier.

It was nothing new. It was a scene I had watched for seven months. Yet somehow this morning it appeared different. God filled me with His heart for Africa and I wept uncontrollably for a half hour. Oh, how he loves the poor. How he weeps with compassion over their suffering. How he longs to heal them and bring joy and prosperity to their land. And oh, how he loves Africa!

As I sought answers about our leaving the poor while the needs remained great, I recorded what God impressed on me that morning:

> As you leave, remember the poor. But follow me. I will have mercy on whom I will have mercy. If I choose to bless you, what is that to you? Guilt is not from me, it is the enemy's way. I love the poor and will look after them. Remember the poor, and be a voice for them.

These refreshing words cleansed my heart and released me to leave freely with His blessing. They clearly confirmed an earlier dream. Feeling as though I had not yet discovered my spiritual destiny, I began to fast and pray. For what purpose had God put me on this earth? Praying on the bow each morning for several months, I asked for a vision to help me understand. I awoke one morning breathless from an extraordinary dream. It clearly revealed His purposes and plans.

The unsettling dream portrayed a despairing view of the poor who were in great danger of dying without Christ. I walked on a sandy beach with thousands of poor people. Suddenly the dark, angry sky signalled danger. I ran quickly to higher ground, and then realized that others remained on the beach oblivious to any danger. Helplessly, I watched as a massive tidal wave buried thousands of people in the mud. I could hear their muffled cries underneath the saturated, sandy floor. The dark skies threatened. I knew that a second tsunami would return to destroy the remaining people. Again no one seemed to sense the impending danger. My physical limitations made it impossible for me to pull people out of the mud. I urgently climbed to a rock calling loudly for the Search and Rescue teams.

High up in strong buildings safe from the dangers, teams merrily engaged in buying and selling. These rescue teams, (the sleeping church) kept fully occupied with financial activities, their fun and entertainment.

"Come and help these people! A tidal wave is coming soon," I called loudly and urgently. Some heard my cries and responded. From a clear position high on a rock, my mission became clear—to use my voice for the poor! It was a dream that would shape my future. A personal mandate from God.

While fighting a daily battle to keep from the enticements of contemporary North American culture, I have sought to be a voice for the poor at every opportunity—to large groups or to an individual waiting in the doctor's office.

I've learned how easy it is to live in this comfortable, bountiful country and chase after its pleasures. While first re-entering our homeland, the strongholds of this nation seemed so apparent. I saw the church in Canada fighting a battle against unbelief, apathy and materialism.

Letting down my spiritual guard, I relaxed immediately since I was no longer on the mission field. A subtle message lured my spirit—*I didn't need to live with a passion for Jesus here at home.* It showed me that I was being lulled into apathy by the enemy.

Also, God seemed hidden by a veil of doubt and unbelief everywhere. For some time, I baffled over my struggle to believe God and sense His presence while living in a supposedly Christian country. I questioned the strength of my faith even after all we had seen and experienced.

Slowly the truth dawned. With so much extravagant wealth, comfort and amusement, it seems there is little need for God in this nation. And what we have is not enough! We are told repeatedly that we need bigger, better and faster. How easily I've found myself drinking from the fountain of materialism and entertainment. An unquenchable thirst fills the soul—one that never satisfies but leaves a desire for more. The sour aftertaste of discontentment follows.

Spare time is quickly filled with movies that titillate our senses, video games of high tech adventures that thrill and kill, computers that support hours of sometimes mindless attention, or amusement parks where a smorgasbord of pleasures await us. Extreme sports, or even the good ol' hockey game, easily become the idols of our soul.

In a book called *Amusing Ourselves to Death*, secular author and communications theorist Neil Postman describes this modern culture's thirst for entertainment:

> There are two ways by which the spirit of a culture may be shriveled. In the first [...] the culture becomes a prison. (The machinery of thought control as it currently operates in scores of countries and on millions of people.) In the second [...] culture becomes a burlesque.[1]

Postman also refers to Aldous Huxley's *Brave New World* in which he teaches:

In the age of advanced technology, spiritual devastation is more likely to come from an enemy with a smiling face than from one whose countenance exudes suspicion and hate.[2]

I heartily concur that the enemy creating spiritual devastation in our Western world owns a smiling face. Our family could easily become amusement addicts needing a constant fix, pushing out our need for solitude and hearing the voice of God. If we've experienced indigestion from our overload of entertainment, we can always tempt our thirst buds with a tour of real estate, shopping malls, furniture or retail outlets, car lots, home, craft or fashion shows, cosmetic and kitchen parties... you name it. We can buy it! But no matter what the price tag, the temporary thrill wears off requiring another possession or replacement of the old.

I understand that wealth, leisure, and entertainment are not wrong in and of themselves. Rather, they are all blessings of God to be enjoyed. It is only when they begin to erode my true purpose as a Christian that I am in danger. We are all called to fulfill God's five purposes for our lives: to worship Him, to fellowship with believers, to grow like Christ, to serve Him in the body of Christ and to be on mission with God in this world.[3] If anything else consumes my time, my thoughts and my lifestyle more than these, my Christian life has lost focus. For this is how we bring glory to God. This is His plan for us. This is what we really live for!

> A life devoted to things is a dead life, a stump; a God-shaped life is a flourishing tree.
>
> Proverbs 11:28 *The Message*

Like a stage of dehydration where the thirst sensation vanishes just before death, eventually I can lose all touch with my spiritual thirst. I forget about the fountain of living water that Jesus described to the woman at the well. I forget how it tastes. I forget how it satisfies. I forget how it gives purpose to my life. Too easily, I find myself drinking at counterfeit fountains. Sometimes God allows circumstances to force my return to His fountain and an understanding of my true purpose for living.

After two months of settling into a public high school in Canada, Brandon, our oldest, came home one day with this interesting observation, "Mom, it's just the same every day in this country. You get up, you go to school, you go to work, you make money and you buy things. That's it! If I didn't have God in my life, it wouldn't be worth living."

These simple words captured the meaninglessness of life that many teens feel in this culture. Brandon, age 14, had spent four years serving the poor and being ruined for the ordinary. He'd been given one of the keys to meaning and purpose in life—that of serving others.

We discovered that our priorities needed to be realigned. Our lives felt like a whirring carousel when we returned to Canada. Due to the high cost of living and our crazy schedules, we often felt like we lived in survival mode. We had to ask ourselves, "Do our full schedules include anything of great significance and eternal value? Do they reflect sacrificial hearts and giving spirits?"

Together we agreed to work monthly in a soup kitchen for the homeless. Preparing and serving them meals regularly forces us to live outside of our own busy schedules and enter the world of the poor in our homeland.

A strictly inward focus can rob our children's minds of spiritual insight and leave them bankrupt. Eventually the meaninglessness of life stares them in the face and they feel ripped off and empty. Is this all there is to the Christian life? As Rick Warren states in his popular book, *The Purpose Driven Life:* "Without a purpose, life is motion without meaning, activity without direction and events without reason. Without a purpose, life is trivial, petty, and pointless."[4]

As we readjusted to life in North America, we became cautious of "amusing ourselves to death" and instead gave ourselves one of the wonderful keys to meaning and purpose in life—serving others. And in doing so, we would still be remembering the poor.

Rich Towards God

Upon re-entry to Canada, it seemed that our children had forgotten the wealth they left behind four years earlier to live on a ship. We all felt the shock upon our return. Schools and parks with myriads of colourful playground equipment awed them. The wastefulness of whole lunches tossed in the garbage appalled them. Talk of computer games they had never heard of set them apart from their peers.

Mega pet stores reminded me of the glorious abundance we share in this land. Advertisements of the latest medical technology for pets saddened me with its reality: animals in this country receive better health care than the majority of people in the world. For me this has become the greatest sign of a wealthy country.

Throughout my life, I've been struck and challenged by Jesus' parable of the rich fool in Luke 11. A man stores up grain and goods for himself, just as we do by our modern retirement savings accounts and bonds. God says, "You fool, this very night your life will be demanded of you. Then what will you get for all you have stored?" That is how it will be for the one who stores up for himself BUT is not "rich towards God." I noted that it does not say "AND is not rich towards God." Scripture does teach us to wisely plan for our future on this earth, but storing up treasure in heaven is paramount. As I enjoy the stores of our wealth on earth, I can easily forget about my heavenly bank account! Hence I find myself loving gold versus loving God!

How can I become rich towards God? There are no heavenly bank statements showing my net worth, no display of assets, RRSP statements or insurance policies by which to measure. The Lord doesn't send me a tally of what I have stored. I am told to simply store up treasure in heaven rather than on earth.

G. Campbell Morgan writes, "Regardless of our net worth, God wants us to be rich. Ah, but that means rich in 'assets' that time cannot tarnish and inflation cannot destroy. It means rich in the assets of righteousness, godliness, faith, love, patience, gentleness. You may possess vast earthly possession but live like a pauper by the one standard that counts for eternity—God's standard."[5]

Since I've spent the majority of my life serving as a mother or volunteer in Christian ministries, I am tempted to complain about the lack of financial payback. I watch other women with money to spend on their children, large homes and spa treatments. Seeds of envy prick at my heart. I forget that I can live with the knowledge that one day my service too will be rewarded, but this kind of reward is *out of this world!*

Every act of mercy or kind word, every sacrifice, and everything we do in the name of the Lord is being recorded in heaven. It is laid up as treasure. The creator of the universe has promised to reward us.

Chapter Twenty Nine

Keith Green, a man whose life and teaching spurred us on to missions, tells the story of a beggar in India.

> This man had been begging all day long and had only a half-cup of rice to show for it. As he was rolling up his begging mat and preparing to leave, he heard the sound of the army approaching. The prince was coming! So he sat down again and waited for the prince to pass by. But as the prince approached, he stopped, climbed down from his elephant, went over to the beggar and asked him for some of his rice.
>
> The beggar stared at him. "What nerve," he thought. "The prince wants my rice. He can afford to buy sacks of rice, and he wants me to give him mine."
>
> Not wanting to refuse the prince, but also not wanting to give up too much of his rice, the beggar counted out three grains of rice and handed them over.
>
> Graciously the prince took the grains of rice and showed them to his head servant. As the prince moved on, the head servant walked over and dropped three gold coins in the beggar's lap. When he saw the coins, he ran after the procession, offering the rest of his rice. But nobody took notice of him.
>
> Of course, if the beggar had known he was going to get a gold coin for every grain of rice he gave, he would gladly have given it all.[6]

The Prince of heaven wants us to exchange all that we cling to for immeasurable riches. Are we going to make the same mistake as this beggar and hold back?

30

Reflections in the Sea

Fear not, for I have redeemed you; I have summoned you by name; you are mine. When you pass through the waters, I will be with you; and when you pass through the rivers, they will not sweep over you. When you walk through the fire, you will not be burned; the flames will not set you ablaze.
Isaiah 43:2

As our family transitioned from our unique lifestyle aboard a hospital ship to the comforts of our homeland, we looked back. I remembered that on a calm day, the glassy ocean mirrored our heads peeking over the bow. Now four years later, we could see new images reflected in the sea. Not only had the children grown taller and their chubby cheeks thinned to more mature angles; not only had their parents acquired deeper facial lines and greying temples; but our new images reflected more than just the passing of time. They reflected a world that expanded from the small town of Seaforth, past our own country and continent to experience new cultures, oceans and continents. They reflected some changes that simply can't be put into words. But the deepest change came from learning to trust in a God who promised to bring us safely through fire and sea. The fires did not burn us, nor the waters rise over us and sweep us away.

Another powerful change resulted from the vast world of those living in poverty! Our family no longer takes for granted the many blessings of living in a developed country. For the privilege of health care—doctors, dentists, optometrists, hospitals and pharmacies—we will always be grateful. In paying taxes, we cherish the luxuries of schools, police, electricity, paved roads, water and sewage systems. Although not easy, we attempt to refrain from complaining and maintain an attitude of thankfulness to God for being such a privileged people. Our new images cannot help but reflect grateful hearts.

Although the poor left their deep imprint on us, sometimes it all seemed too hard—too difficult for our family to carry on sacrificing and struggling on a ship for the poor. But unlike television, we couldn't just flick the channel to avoid seeing sorrowful images of the poor. The poor lived beyond our porthole, gripping our hearts and holding us captive. How could we carry on with our lives as before? Impossible. The poor had changed each of us. When self-pity knocked on our cabin door, we remembered how the poor lived in contrast to us on the Mercy Ship.

When it became hard for our family to live in a small cabin

Chapter Thirty

space, we remembered that a Trinidad family's home was a dark, leaky goat shack with a dirt floor. No electricity. No pictures on the walls. No shower or toilet.

When it grew tiring to walk the length of a football field to the laundry room for our scheduled time slot, we remembered Josephine, who carried water from a well. She used plastic bowls for washing clothes, and then laid each garment on the sun-parched red earth to dry.

When it felt laborious having to unfold our futon couch into a bed every evening, and fold it back again in the morning, we remembered our port security guards who had no bed, just a flea-infested mat on the dirty concrete.

When it was distressing to be sick with tropical infections, diarrhea, and living with the threat of malaria, we remembered Maurice: a young boy nurses put out on the steps of a local hospital because he had no more money for medical care. He died.

When we grew weary of lining up daily in the overcrowded dining room to get our food, we remembered. Empty stomachs of the blind, the limbless, and the begging children continually called out to us from street corners and crowded market places.

When it hurt to see our children homesick, living away from grandparents and cousins, we remembered. Many are the orphans of Africa. Some have been sold by parents as slaves in the black market. Abandoned and homeless.

When it became difficult to work as volunteers having to fully rely on God for provision of sponsorship through churches, family and friends, we remembered. For many Africans, it was pure daily survival. No word for "future" existed in many of their languages and Voodoo gods didn't provide.

When it was sad to leave for home and resettle in our rich country of Canada, we remembered that for the West Africans, Africa WAS home. A nation still bound in the clutches of suffering and poverty.

Yes, many things felt hard, but we will always remember the poor of Africa. We will be forever grateful for the incredible journey God led our family on to reach out to them with the two handed expression of the gospel—one hand to bring physical healing and one to offer spiritual hope.

On the morning of our departure from the ship, friends crowded in the reception foyer waiting to say farewell. Bags bulging with all our earthly possessions and one African drum in tow, the Meyers' family trundled down the gangway one final time. We turned again to hug tearful friends in the crowd. At such a time, words seemed futile. Moments before leaving, suddenly the deafening ship's horn blasted numerous times. We looked up to Lido Deck to see Captain Clem in uniform saluting our departure. It was an unforgettable gesture of honour.

Like the others onboard, we were just an ordinary family who dared to dream of sailing to the poor. Ten feet had travelled the globe by ship, airplane, train, Land Rover and taxi. The journey spanned three continents and 16 countries. Brimming with adventure, rife with hardship and danger, overflowing with blessing, the journey had been worth it all! With so great a need in the world, how could we have done anything less?

Afterglow

In July of 2001, our family exchanged brass portholes for curtained windows, our blue ocean view for green grass, lush woods and brilliant flower gardens. Our new home is tucked away in Waterdown, Ontario—named after its waterfalls. The lane connects to a road that winds over the Niagara escarpment, and leads to Lake Ontario. An eight-minute coast downhill takes us directly to this Great Lake. This vast body of water can almost feel like the ocean, but the freshwater waves are lighter and smaller. As Bruce and I walk the stony shores and gaze at the sapphire, sparkling waters and distant horizon, we share an ache and a longing.

The dream grows more distant behind us and leaves an ache in our hearts. The longing to sail the mighty oceans will always remain with us. But the longing to reach distant shores and touch the lives of the poor with His love and mercy is stronger than ever. Yet above all this lays the greatest longing of all—to someday look into the eyes and gaze at the nail-scarred Hands of the Master Potter, the One we have loved and trusted with our lives.

In a friend's home sits a fascinating fountain art piece designed for relaxation. Water trickles smoothly over a small cascade of rocks. White pillared candles rise and unify within the fountain. It is starkly pure and lovely in its simplicity of white.

Mark's casual comment about the fountain captured me and continues to draw me to the piece every time I visit, "I like the combination of fire and water."

Fire and water are powerful images symbolic of purification and cleansing. Apart from these symbols of baptism for believers, God often leads us on a personal, unique journey through fire and water. Unlike the relaxing fountain art piece, the journey isn't always serene.

Scorching flames burned and purged away impurities and unholiness in our lives as our health was struck and dreams died. In their resurrection, hope had been restored. While at sea, healing washed over us like soothing waves of mercy. By taking us through fire and sea, God had shaped us into vessels of mercy to bring hope and healing to the poor. Over the four years onboard we witnessed thousands of lives changed by hope and healing, including our own! The voyage between Seaforth and Waterdown had shown us our own reflections in the sea.

Mark and Sherry's living room is welcoming, soothing and relaxing. The pillared candle flames flicker, the water trickles endlessly. As I sit sharing a cup of tea with Sherry, I now too, bathe peacefully in the warm afterglow of His fire and water in my life. I will savour this season, at least for a time, until the next big wave comes along.

Chapter Thirty

We went through fire and water, but you brought us to a place of abundance.
Psalm 66:12

Notes:

Chapter 3 – Tests in the Wilderness
Jill Austin, *The Last Days Magazine*. "In The Hands of the Master Potter" (Lindale, TX: Last Days Ministries, 1992), 10. The structure of the clay pot stages was developed and adapted from this article.

Chapter 4 – Soul Thirst
Selwyn Hughes, *Everyday with Jesus*. Nov/Dec Issue, "Wilderness Experience" (Surrey, England: CWR, Waverley Abbey House, 1993), December 22, 1993
2 Ibid, December 21, 1993 "Law of Opposites"

Chapter 5 – Silence in the Crib
Selwyn Hughes, *Everyday with Jesus*. Nov/Dec Issue, "Wilderness Experience" (Surrey, England: CWR, Waverley Abbey House, 1993), December 23, 1993 "Law of Opposites"

Chapter 7 – Beauty from Ashes
Oswald Chambers, *My Utmost For His Highest* (Grand Rapids, MI: Discovery House Publishers, 1992), February 10

Chapter 8 – Currier & Ives
CE Chaffin, TS Eliot, *Four Quartets*, IV. Fire vs. Fire 1/30/06 Retrieved April 24, 2006 http://www.melicreview.com/current/chaffin%20essay.htm
2 Jill Austin, *The Last Days Magazine*. "In The Hands of the Master Potter" (Lindale, TX: Last Days Ministries, 1992), 16

Chapter 9 – Embers of a Dream
Loren Cunningham, *Is That Really You God?* (Seattle, WA, YWAM Publishing, 1984), Appendix
2 Oswald, Chambers, *My Utmost For His Highest* (Grand Rapids, MI: Discovery House Publishers, 1992), January 19

Notes

Chapter 17 – Steel Scars
Anastasis Communications Department, Mercy Ships Fleet Reports November 1 -15, 2000 Sierra Leone and Benin, News Flash – Anastasis "Bump" Damages Lifeboat, 1
2 Ibid

Chapter 22 – Clay Vessels of Mercy
Oswald Chambers, *My Utmost For His Highest* (Grand Rapids, MI: Discovery House Publishers, 1992), November 11

Chapter 27 – Mercy Hands
Don Stephens, *Mandate for Mercy* (Seattle, WA: YWAM Publishing, 1992), 24

Chapter 29 – Remember the Poor
Neil Postman, *Amusing Ourselves to Death* (Toronto, ON: Penquin Books,1985) 155
2 Ibid
3 Rick Warren, *The Purpose Driven Life*, (Grand Rapids, MI: Zondervan, 2002) 303
4 Ibid, 30
5 G. Campbell Morgan, *Compass Devotional Magazine*, Mercy Ships
6 Keith Green, *A Cry in the Wilderness* (Nashville, TN: Sparrow Press, 1993), 138

photo acknowledgements

Photo Credits: Mercy Ships International
- Surgery onboard
- International Christian School in Benin – 2001
- Screening Day in Benin
- Mutala Before Surgery
- Mutala After
- Malik Before Surgery
- Malik After
- Three year-old Cavilla
- Cavilla's village
- m/v *Anastasis*
- "Sailing is serene, marvellous beyond words."

Special thanks to Sharon Nelson at Mercy Ships International for her resourceful efforts in searching out photos from the archives.

> Mercy Ships images may not be used to represent or promote another organization without the expressed written permission obtained from the VP of Communications. Mercy Ships images may not be altered if the alteration results in a material change in either the content or the message of the original image. Copyright © 2006 Mercy Ships International All rights reserved.

Photo Credit: Lynn Toney
- Meyers family on shores of Benin – 2000

Photo Credit: Bruce Meyers
- Brandon, Chadwick and Jillian on Promenade Deck
- Jillian at the Sisters of Charity Orphanage
- Painted Porthole on C-deck
- Damage to wing during "touching" accident
- Widow Josephine in front of her hovel

Photo Credit: Debbie Blades
Author, Back Cover

Acknowledgement: Book Cover original design concept by Chadwick Meyers

The author appreciates the journey you embarked on by reading this story and welcomes your comments. To order more books or to arrange for a speaking engagement, please send correspondence to:

Marilyn Meyers
P.O. Box 545,
Waterdown, ON
CANADA
L0R 2H0

Or visit:
www.fireandsea.com

CASTLE QUAY BOOKS

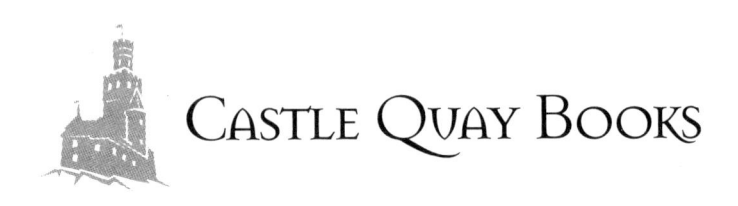

OTHER CASTLE QUAY TITLES INCLUDE:
Walking Towards Hope
The Chicago Healer
Seven Angels for Seven Days
Making Your Dreams Your Destiny
The Way They Should Go
The Defilers
Jesus and Caesar
Jason Has Been Shot!
The Cardboard Shack Beneath the Bridge - **NEW!**
Keep On Standing - **NEW!**
To My Family - **NEW!**

BayRidge Books titles:
Counterfeit Code: Answering The Da Vinvi Code Heresies
Father to the Fatherless: The Charles Mulli Story
Wars Are Never Enough: The Joao Matwawana Story
More Faithful Than We Think

For more information and to explore the rest of our titles visit
www.castlequaybooks.com